An introduction to Self-Care using inversion
as a central Wellness tool

The
Inversion
Revolution

Beyond Back Pain to Wellness

by Michael J. McKay L.M.T.

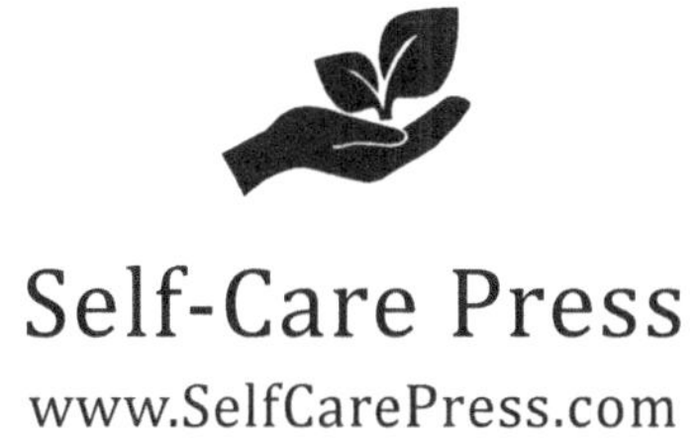

Self-Care Press
www.SelfCarePress.com

The Inversion Revolution
Beyond Back Pain to Wellness

Published by
Self-Care Press
August 2017

© 2017 by Michael J. McKay L.M.T.
All rights reserved.

Printed in the United States of America

Self-Care Press
202 South Second St
Fairfield, Iowa 52556
www.SelfCarePress.com

ISBN: 978-0-9826615-2-9

Dedication

For Dawn

You taught me that Self-Care is not Alone-Care.
Your loving touch has healed me most of all.

TABLE OF CONTENTS

FOREWORD

THE INVERSION REVOLUTION STARTS HERE

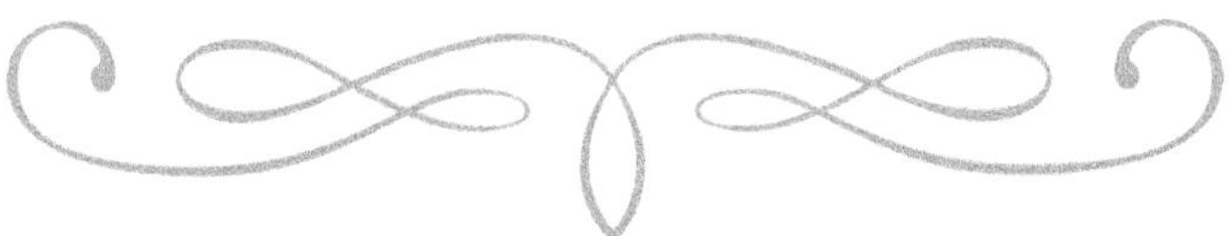

If you're reading this you're likely to be either in pain or have a loved one who's in pain.

What you or they are looking for – first and foremost – is relief.

Relief from pain is what led me to inversion, in my case desperately needing relief from crippling back pain and an impending surgery.

And I found it. Something shifted and frankly I was lucky.

But can inversion offer a broader range of benefits beyond pain relief? Can it offer *more?*

I initially used my early version Gravity Pal® low angle inversion table and found the pain relief I desperately needed. But then I found *more*. As time went on I discovered a method of using inversion that improved my quality of life in ways I wasn't expecting. I now call these Wellness "side-benefits."

The real surprise was when these Wellness side-benefits started to be reported to me by other people, by those who had purchased my Gravity Pal® low angle inversion tables. These people, also, were not looking for these side-benefits. But they came. Not the same ones to everyone. Some people reported clearer thinking, some improved energy, and so on.

But it was clear that something else, something deeper was happening, a general quality of life improvement seemed to be the consistent report. One gentleman reported a less-droopy eyelid, something that had bothered him all his life. Others reported improvements in their digestion that they weren't initially looking for.

This fascinated me. My primary motivation to manufacture my Gravity Pal® low angle inversion tables came from my finding *relief*.

I had found significant pain and compression relief from using them and wanted to share that kind of relief with others. Once my massage clients saw this shift in me, they asked me to make them one. And so we started.

But along the way it became clear that we'd started something that has a larger potential. I now believe we're at the beginning point of an *Inversion Revolution*.

This revolution started with an idea and an observation.

The idea behind this revolution is that the <u>method</u> of using inversion is more important than simply looking at inversion alone.

The observation: when the right method is used many additional side-benefits can potentially be experienced. These side benefits indicate a broader impact of inversion than pain and compression relief. They point to many healthful physiological effects happening – all at the same time.

Going Upside Down is Obvious and Incomplete

Inversion seemed so intuitive – so obvious to me. Turn myself upside down and let gravity decompress the problem I was having. Obvious. Simple ... and incomplete. I never thought to think or ask anyone if there was a better – or best – way to invert. *"Give Me Relief"* was all I could think about.

Once I achieved a small measure of relief I was still far away from celebrating Wellness in my life. I struggled and along the way I found many tools, each with their own value, but I kept coming back to inversion. And the more I used it, the more I began to appreciate it as a tool that most people simply did not know how to use.

I would talk to people about inversion and they would – over and over again – tell me that they had purchased a high angle inversion table they were no longer using, or had never used! *"It's collecting dust in my garage"* was a frequent comment. *"It scared me"* was the other most frequent comment.

I started researching these tables and found they all had similar instructions and warnings. They commonly told people to start off slowly – at a lower angle and shorter times on it – and to gradually "work up to" higher angles and longer times on it, most commonly 15 or more minutes. I asked myself the question – *"what would be the lowest angle and the shortest time where inversion might be useful?"*

I researched the history of inversion and found that it crosses cultures and can be traced back thousands of years to ancient Greece and India. Throughout the centuries inversion has been used for pain relief as well as for training elite athletes in modern-day gymnastics.

It is said that Hippocrates, circa 400 BC, witnessed two people lashing some poor soul to a ladder and turning them upside down. Inversion was obvious – and primitive – then, so much so that these people didn't ask Hippocrates for *"a better way to invert."*

Neither is there a record of Hippocrates volunteering them any advice as to how to – maybe – make inversion more effective.

Amazingly, even to this day, there has been virtually no research on a *method* that can more effectively use inversion to bring relief. Also, there has been zero research on the other potential Wellness side-benefits that can come from a proper method of inversion.

No one has taken the time or put forth the effort to look deeply into the human physiology and ask the questions that could hopefully make inversion a more effective Self-Care tool.

This book about the *Inversion Revolution* is a starting point that hopefully will spur objective scientific research on inversion. You'll hear me invite researchers over and over to "look here" and I'll present why they should do so.

The *Inversion Revolution* Looks Beyond Relief to Wellness

We want more than relief. We want more than just getting our heads above water and feeling grateful we haven't drowned. However, if relief was all that inversion delivered that would be just fine.

But what if inversion can deliver more? Can inversion be useful as a tool for a better state of health and Wellness?

I believe it can.

I have experienced that people using the right *method* of inversion may also notice a number of "side-benefits" they weren't looking for. The proper method not only can provide relief for many people but can add significant other health benefits, such as:

- ❖ Enhanced Mental Clarity
- ❖ Improved Energy
- ❖ Reduced Stress
- ❖ Faster Recovery from Exercise
- ❖ ... and even Healthier Skin

The *Inversion Revolution* looks beyond simple compression and back pain relief to celebrating Wellness, to using inversion as a key Self-Care tool to achieve improved overall health.

We will examine a method where we can harness gravity to not only assist healing – and bring relief – but to potentially be a <u>central</u> Wellness tool. Inversion is only one tool, but I believe it can be as important as nutrition, exercise and good sleep. Inversion – done properly – can be a basic part of living better.

I believe there will come a day when inversion tables – used properly – will be as common as chairs and people will routinely use them for Wellness and regaining balance.

Inversion Alone is Not Enough

Over the past thirty years millions of people have sought relief and thought inversion was a way to get it.

Every one of these people was presented the obvious: gravity might help them. I contend that none of these people were presented two fundamental things that would allow them to discover how to best use inversion. And it is the lack of understanding of these two things that has kept inversion – until now – an incomplete tool. Inversion *alone* is not enough.

These two things are:
1. The body has a natural wiring that protects us when we encounter surprise events – we tense up. It is important to NOT trigger that tension trigger when we invert.

2. The body's primary requirement for Balance is something inversion – when properly done – can help gain and regain.

Up until now our natural "Startle Reflex" has been ignored. Unless done properly, the human nervous system may think that inversion is a *threat*. **The body's natural reaction to instability is to tense up in readiness to defend itself!**

A method of inversion had to be developed to keep the body from reacting in that protective way. Inversion alone may trigger the body to actually tense up more – precisely the opposite of the first goal of inversion: to release tension.

Inversion is not one of our normal "vector relationships" with gravity. Normally we have four: Standing, Sitting, Walking and Lying Down. Three of these relationships with gravity are vertical and one is horizontal. None of them are at an angle and none of them are lying backward with our head at a downward angle.

The body has a natural reaction when it encounters fear, pain and instability. It is alternatively called both the "Startle Reflex" and "Muscle Guarding" and both mean the same thing – the body tenses up automatically and involuntarily.

As you will learn, what is of key importance is to NOT trigger this reflex during inversion. **Fortunately, I have created a way to invert so that the nervous system feels safe and secure, which allows inversion to provide the relaxation we are seeking.**

This natural tendency that we do NOT want to trigger is totally overlooked in the general discussion on inversion. The other most overlooked aspect of our human nervous system is the role of "Balance" in our Health and Wellness.

Balance and regaining balance, as we will discuss, is fundamental to our health. It is why we sleep and why we take in nutrition. Balance and regaining balance is how we both avoid disease and heal from disease. If inversion is used properly it can be a godsend to helping us gain and regain this most essential state on a daily basis.

In presenting these two points it is obvious we need to cover some basic groundwork and agree on some basic terms. We can't just bandy about the terms Wellness, Health and Balance.

We have to agree about what "Health" is and what "Disease" is. You will come to understand that this has been the subject of considerable controversy. We will resolve this by presenting a practical definition of "Health" and "Disease" that is empowering to us and each member of our Self-Care team.

I will present to you the "Six Stages of Disease" which will explain the vital role of "Balance."

You will learn the Wellness Dance. There are four dance steps to Wellness. You'll learn what they are and how to flow between them.

Based on this you will get a historic perspective on inversion and, most importantly, a beginning appreciation of why and how the *Gravity Pal Inversion Method™* works.

Once you have this background you'll be ready to build your own tool-kit which is one of the most important parts of this book.

Inversion for Self-Care

As mentioned earlier, inversion has caught the attention of millions of people, many of whom swear it helps them.

Yet the Mayo Clinic has chosen, so far, to only evaluate *high angle* inversion as a method for back pain relief and has – appropriately –

said it is not safe for everyone. I support the Mayo Clinic's warning to the public that high angle approaches may be unsafe. This is simply being responsible about it.

It is obvious that many people are intimidated, even scared – for good reasons – of high angle inversion options and yet, until this book, there has been no public discussion of what constitutes a more *responsible* approach to inversion.

But this is not a book to completely bash high angle inversion as an option. Many people find great value in using the higher angle inversion tables – in spite of the appropriate warnings presented by the Mayo Clinic.

I am the developer and manufacturer of Gravity Pal® <u>low angle</u> inversion tables and have an admitted prejudice that low angle inversion is a better option than high angle inversion tables for many – and perhaps even most people.

I'm obviously committed to this view and am "all in:" putting my money and my family's financial future where my beliefs are. And I speak from experience. Daily sessions of low angle inversion on my Gravity Pal® are central to my pain relief and management process and have literally changed my life. In this book I will make my unapologetic case for why I believe our low angle approach is better than higher angle options for many reasons.

However, let me be clear, *it is the proper method of inversion itself* that I believe will assist people to live better. Some people can tolerate higher angles and some people may even prefer them. Discovering a responsible way and method to invert has never before been discussed.

The unique method of inversion I've developed, the *Gravity Pal Inversion Method™*, including the angle, the duration of a session and the frequency of sessions – will be presented as well as why this method dramatically improves the effectiveness of inversion.

The book concludes with a discussion about the *Self-Care Revolution* that has already arrived and I believe will only become a stronger force in the years to come.

The Inversion Revolution & The Self-Care Revolution

Western medicine, in particular, has a wonderful opportunity to partner with each individual's journey even as more and more responsibility transfers from the physician as "Health Care Provider" to the individual as "Self-Care General Contractor." This transfer of responsibility from doctor to patient is at the core of the Self-Care Revolution and will be expanded upon and discussed throughout the book.

Inversion, *responsible* inversion, I believe will be appreciated in the years to come as a central component of Self-Care. I believe that low angle inversion, experienced in 1 to 3 minute increments and repeated 2 or 3 times per day can have a wide range of positive impacts for a broad range of the population whether young, old, infirm or in great health.

The testimonials and stories from enthusiastic Gravity Pal® users I will share are only a small sample of those regularly received.

Not only do we hear claims of relief from back, hip, shoulder and neck pain, we consistently hear from people who report what we can only call Wellness benefits. These include thinking more clearly, having more energy, sleeping better, enjoying better digestion and several other happy results.

These additional benefits – leading people toward a greater experience of Wellness – have been a major inspiration for writing this book.

Why do these reported results happen? Is it a placebo effect? Certainly one cannot dismiss that possibility out of hand since some studies on placebo effects have shown positive results in up to 30% of control groups who receive nothing at all.[1]

But what if these positive effects from our unique method of using low angle inversion are not a placebo effect? What if these effects are due to physical reality – as I believe they are – rather than psychological beliefs?

Personally, as you will read in my story, I don't think I avoided an imminent back surgery because the relief from crippling back pain I obtained from using my low angle inversion table was "all in my head" – or even potentially in my head.

Neither do I believe that people tell me they *"miss their daily Gravity Pal® sessions"* when they have to be away from them – simply because they have been experiencing a placebo.

Nevertheless, we live in the scientific age and anything that is good and repeatable by most people should be able to withstand the critically harsh scrutiny of objective scientific testing.

I believe there are sound scientific reasons why people are experiencing the many positive results using Gravity Pal® low angle inversion tables presented here.

---

[1] The placebo effect is a controversial subject where some researchers argue it does not exist at all. The best article I have found discussing this subject is by Brissonnet, Jean, *Placebo, Are You There?*, February 24, 2015, https://sciencebasedmedicine.org/placebo-are-you-there/

Throughout the book I repeat an invitation to researchers to objectively evaluate these reports, and outline reasonable scientific theories I hope will assist serious researchers in those efforts. I want to encourage objective scientific research on inversion and its effects and it is my sincere hope that professional researchers will respond, obtain the funding, conduct the studies and publish the results.

I'm well aware it's not valid to say that science has "proved" this or that, in the same way that physics can never reach Absolute Zero. Mostly, science tries to disprove a thesis. If it cannot disprove a finding one way then it tries to disprove it another way. The more times science fails to disprove something the more "certain" science – begrudgingly – allows there to be, maybe, a cause-effect relationship.

Ironically, even though there is a very long history of inversion going back to before the time of Hippocrates, there are very few scientific studies on inversion in general and there are *none* I know of on low angle inversion that can be found. Also, completely missing in the scientific literature are any studies of the long term *cumulative* effects of regular, short duration sessions of high or low inversions.

I say to the (appropriately) skeptical researchers – *"Bring it on – please."*

To the public I offer a suggestion: give low angle inversion with a Gravity Pal® a try. It's a low cost option that may take you, like it has for me and many others, beyond back pain to Wellness.

Michael McKay
Founder Gravity Pal®
www.GravityPal.com

CHAPTER 1

MY STORY – HOW I OVERCAME A LIFE OF BACK PAIN

My personal search to alleviate severe pain
is how the Gravity Pal® story began.

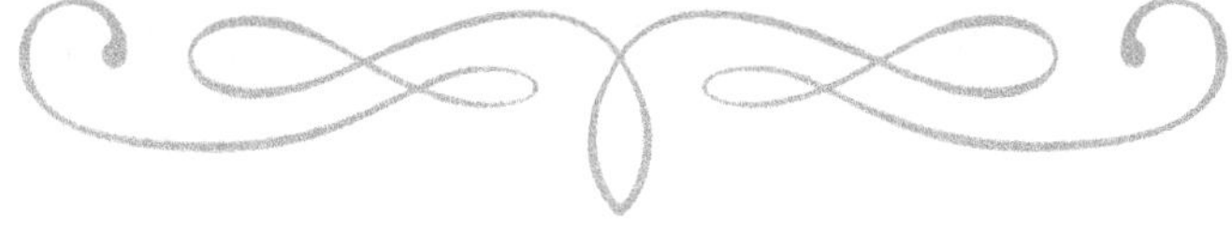

I remember even as a kid having back pain but I dismissed it to youthful sports injuries and the occasional weekend warrior overuse. But I was wrong, very wrong. Many years later, my doctor told me the root cause of my lifelong back pain problem was a congenital birth defect where the facets in my lower back area had not developed correctly in the first place. Who knew?

So, one day in 2000 at age 49, while merely getting out of a booth in a restaurant after lunch the top of my spine at L4 slid forward from my lower spine at L5 thus severely pinching and stretching the nerves bundled there. The shocking pain in my back and legs was breathtaking and indescribable. I couldn't walk more than a few steps before I had to stop and I couldn't stand for more than several seconds at a time. It was all I could do to get home that day and see straight.

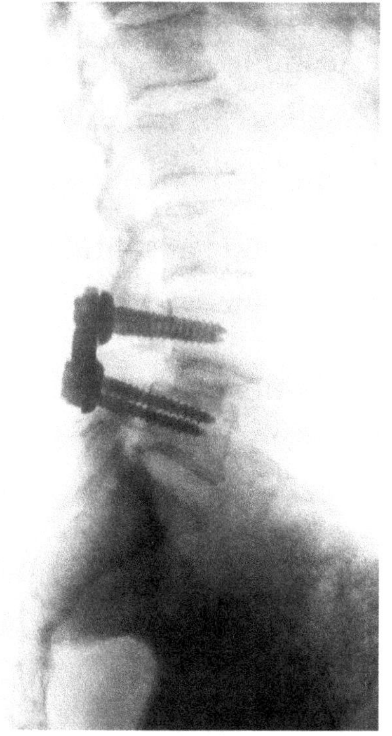

X-Ray of my spine after my surgery

The term *"brought to my knees"* was, for me, what actually happened.

After reviewing the MRI, the neurosurgeons said I had a condition called *"spondylolisthesis."* They quickly set me up for spinal fusion surgery and I thank God they did. This condition can quickly wreck the nerves and they wanted to move fast. But, unfortunately for me, it was not fast enough.

Even though the surgically installed titanium "cage" stabilized my spine, extensive nerve damage had been done. I was left with intense 24/7 pain down both of my legs. I came to appreciate many different kinds of pain: biting, burning, sharp, stabbing, shooting, tearing, piercing, throbbing, and aching. It was a tough time and a very fearful one for me and my family.

One compassionate doctor told me that this was called *"peripheral neuropathy,"* that there was no cure, and that all I could do was to manage it with (a lifetime of) prescription drugs. He kindly said that I should simply "shake hands with my pain."

I said, *"No thank you"* and that is when my real journey began.

I decided to become an expert in how to not only minimize pain, but to overcome it.

My journey has led me to extensively study and engage in many excellent modalities and activities that have assisted me to become *mostly* pain free today. These include Pilates, Rolfing, Gyrotonics, Myofascial Release Therapy, Five-Element Acupuncture, Zero Balancing, chiropractic, massage, weight training, yoga, rock climbing and, now, low angle inversion with Gravity Pal®.

As with many journeys, mine has many chapters and adventures. I did not know (and do not remember anyone telling me) in 2001 that the surgical fusion of spinal vertebrae together can require OTHER spinal fusion surgeries later on, due to the additional stress put on the other nearby joints by the initial surgery. Holy cow!

I did not know that it is very common to later need to fuse the vertebrae above and below the original spot. So, several years after my initial surgery, in spite of all of my efforts and improvements, I found myself suffering again and scheduled for a second back surgery. While at what I would call my peak recovery fitness level I was simply putting something in my car and *BAM* I was on my knees again.

It was pretty depressing.

I had worked so hard and made so much progress. I went from barely being able to stand in the kitchen to make a meal in 2001, to rock climbing in Yosemite, California in 2006. My biggest dream in 2001 was to be able to stand and walk long enough to take my (then) 7-year-old daughter to Disney World. Only a few years later I felt I had beat it and had truly transformed my life.

Truth is, I *had* transformed my life. But I now had to overcome a new challenge, a setback, a new obstacle that I did not see coming.

But just then a fortunate thing happened.

About a week before this new surgery, while I was using an early version of Gravity Pal® – which was the only thing that was giving me any relief at all – I felt something *positively* shift in my back and felt much better upon getting up off of it. It was a delightful surprise, but I was still wary.

I called my neurosurgeon and we postponed that surgery, first week by week then bi-weekly for a couple of months, then we simply put it off altogether.

It was then I knew that I had to further develop and bring Gravity Pal® and low angle inversion out into the world.

While I cannot promise anyone will have the same results as I did, I do know that Self-Care is what is working for me and my Gravity Pal® is a big part of that equation.

Years ago, my wife and I – together – went back to school and became licensed massage therapists and obtained advanced training as integrative bodywork therapists. Our original motivation was so that we could take better care of each other as we were getting older.

But now I had a new motivation; I started to more deeply study. I wanted to REALLY understand what had happened to me and to figure out how to better treat myself to have the best level of health possible. I wanted to understand as deeply as possible how low angle inversion could benefit me and others.

As I studied the long history from over 2000 years ago and many recent invention ideas since 1890, I found that inversion as a therapy is a very old idea, and that there have been many, oftentimes questionable ways that it has been attempted throughout history. Significantly, the recent infatuation with high angle approaches has been so successfully promoted that the public and even the Mayo Clinic equate inversion as a potential therapy with "high angle."

This is a mistake.

For me and many others, higher angle options are simply too scary and impractical for multiple reasons. I wanted something different from high angle inversion that was not scary, that didn't take 15 minutes, did not require a spotter or person to make sure I did not get stuck upside down.

Instead, I wanted something that was not scary yet effective, that was both quick to do and convenient for my life.

I knew I needed something with which I could travel and was therefore lightweight and portable.

It was obvious that high angle inversion options were not portable.

Mine has been a journey of humility, setbacks and exciting discoveries. Today I am pain-free most of the time. I use my Gravity Pal® 2 to 3 times every day for only 1 to 3 minutes at a time. Occasionally I use it only once or twice in a day and occasionally I use it for only a single minute as a session. Over and over again I have been impressed with how a little of this technology goes a long, long way in providing me with immediate compression relief.

After several months of consistent, daily use I started to discover something else – that regularly using my Gravity Pal® on a daily basis was improving other areas of my health I wasn't even looking for.

I started to notice that my thinking was becoming clearer. Believe me, after dealing with persistently high levels of pain for many years it was a real contrast to be able to think more clearly.

After numerous other Gravity Pal® users reported that they, too had started to experience greater mental clarity, my wife and I started to research how using a Gravity Pal® might contribute to that experience.

For now, even though these reports are very exciting and we think there are sound scientific reasons why there is a connection to regularly using a Gravity Pal®, all we can provide are anecdotal reports.

If anyone reading this is a legitimate scientific researcher working through an accredited university or research institute who would like to conduct objective tests on this phenomenon, please contact me. I would like to see if these reports can be objectively verified and would be happy to supply, free of charge and without restrictions or any request for attribution, the low angle inversion tables needed to conduct this research.

I started this journey searching for relief from debilitating back pain. Many people – too many people – today are searching for that same relief. As a tool, Gravity Pal® started out as a re-discovery and further refinement of the ancient human quest to escape the compressive effects of gravity. Along the way the bigger surprise has been to discover a tool that appears to have a broad spectrum of Wellness benefits that I wasn't even looking for.

Now I look beyond my initial need for back pain relief which I happily manage every day. Now I look forward to better health and a better quality of life in many different ways – much more than I thought possible only a few short years ago.

CHAPTER 2

I DISCOVERED AN EMPOWERED MODEL OF HEALTH & WELLNESS

What is Health?
A Short History and a New Definition

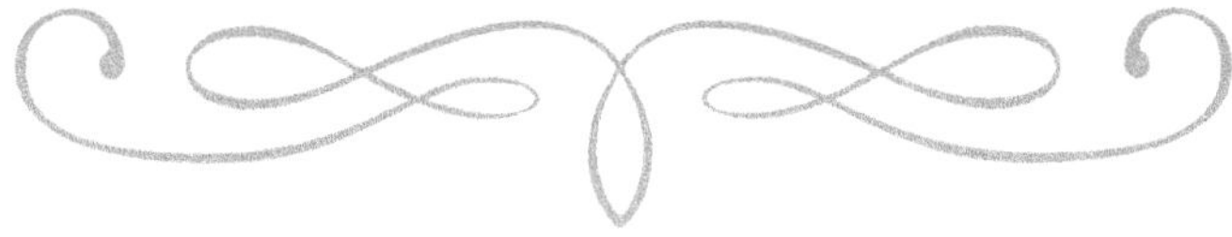

What is Health? What is Disease?

It may be shocking to hear but Western healthcare <u>does not</u> provide a precise and widely accepted definition of health. How can this be?

Even though healthcare occupies 18% of GDP in the United States and a large portion of most Western economies, there is considerable disagreement, confusion – and downright denial – over defining the word health.

And this has consequences for all of us, physicians and patients alike.

On the surface, such a definition might seem obvious but a battle has been raging for hundreds of years over defining this simple word.

Let's start with the common dictionary definition which states:

"Health is simply the absence of disease."

If that is so, how do we account for healthy blind people who are totally functional and maybe superlatively productive in the world? Are they unhealthy?

And how are we to think about elderly athletes who run marathons even though they may have pacemakers or may be dealing with any number of health challenges?

Or do we accept the 1949 definition of health from the World Health Organization which states:

"Health is a state of complete physical, mental, and social well-being, and not merely the absence of disease or infirmity."

The problem here is the word "complete." When health is defined as a state of *"complete physical, mental and social well-being"* it makes it hard to believe that anyone is healthy![2]

A New Definition of Health and Disease

We live in the real world and must take into account that everyone has some kind of challenge, large or small, mental or physical – and that these vary in intensity from time to time.

Some of us have a chronic condition and yet we are able to be productive and find great satisfaction in our lives – and here is the important part – in spite of the challenges we face.

Therefore, I'll offer these definitions originated by medical commentator, Dr. Michel Accad,

Health is when a person's physical and mental conditions allow the pursuit of his or her chosen ends. Disease, then, is the absence of health.[3]

What are "chosen ends?" They are whatever we may want to do at any given moment.

- ❖ If we want to garden – we can do it
- ❖ If we want to take a walk – we can do it
- ❖ If we want to run a marathon or rock climb at age 66 – well, maybe we can do it if we work hard enough

---

[2] How should we define health? http://www.bmj.com/content/343/bmj.d4163 accessed January 18, 2017

[3] Dr. Michel Accad, MD, blogs at *http://alertandoriented.com/* and is highly recommended. I liberally refer to a lecture by Dr. Accad which you can hear at: *https://mises.org/library/dr-michel-accad-can-austrian-economics-save-medicine.*

Notice even a young person may not be healthy enough by this definition to play, say, middle linebacker in the NFL. Notice also that health can be developed and improved to allow one to – maybe – rock climb at age 66 or beyond.

Your chosen end may not be practical – today or ever. But then again, if you can pretty much do everything you may desire to do, then you are healthy – enough.

How we answer this question: "What is Health?" – is critical. We must define both health and disease in order to meaningfully discuss what Wellness is.

How Did This Debate Get Started?
A Brief History of the Definition of Health

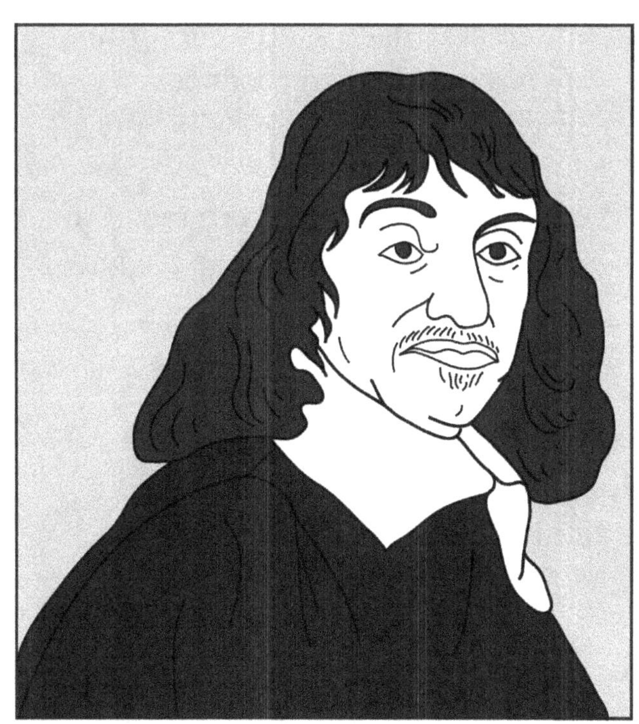

In the West we can thank René Descartes (1596 AD to 1650 AD) who, in the early days of the scientific revolution, proposed the machine concept of the human body.

At that time Descartes's proposal was a radical departure from earlier ideas that humans had what were called essences and natures. Instead, Descartes said the human body was a complex assembly of parts that moved mechanically according to physical laws. He said these mechanical parts are under the control of a separate human soul which acts like a *ghost in a machine.*

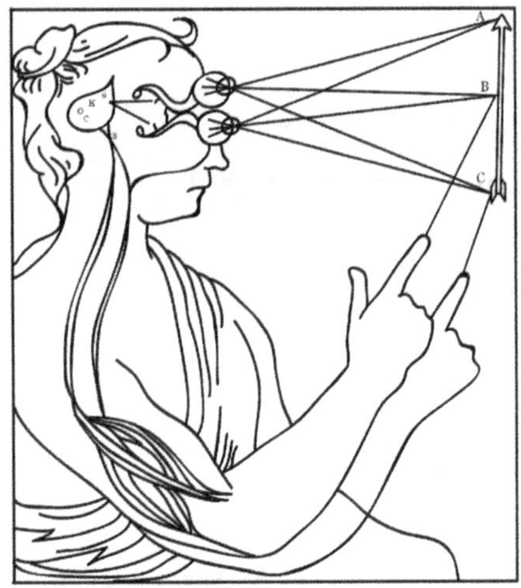

Descartes's model of the human body as a machine proved very useful. In the centuries that followed it facilitated many new and important scientific discoveries.

Organisms were revealed to be made of basic material parts that could be described in detail and closely observed to act on and interact with each other according to physical laws to produce predictable biological behaviors.

Research advanced and showed increasing promise. As a result the machine model was increasingly adopted by scientists on a wide scale.

Medical Licensing Laws
Formally Institutionalized the Machine Model
in Medical Education

Since the early days of the 20th century, Western medicine primarily focuses on the physical pieces of the body and physical and chemical reactions and interactions. What has largely been ignored is any evaluation on the "Whole Person" level.

Also, since 1900, economic factors have dramatically improved, resulting in a burgeoning middle class with dramatically longer life spans for the average person.

In other words, at the same time Western medicine was embracing the "parts" and ignoring the "whole," people were living longer – or we could say – surviving longer.

Because their external circumstances were much improved over the eras of famine and mass diseases, people were interested in and looking forward to living longer than ever before.

Now, for the first time in human history, the general population (in the West) *expects* to live for decades after retirement while surrounded by comforts and conveniences.

The medical profession bloomed in the 20th century. But it did so based on an incomplete model and an incomplete definition of health. We are, after all, more than mere machines.

Throughout the middle and later years of the 20th century the West became more aware of Eastern models, like Ayurveda from India and Chinese medicine, which focus beyond the machine model and include an understanding of the energy systems in the body.

Many in Western medicine, meanwhile, ignored or strongly discouraged acknowledging the energy aspects of the body; even going so far as to denigrate these "alternative" forms of medicine altogether. We continue see some of that tendency even today.

Why?

Models.

We humans use models, which we also can call *paradigms,* every day to decide which bits of information we should pay attention to and which we should ignore. We can't help it; it's the way we we're wired to think.[4]

Even though it was flawed, it was a great boon to think of the body as a machine. No one can deny this. However, once the machine model became a shared paradigm *of how we should think* by a number of prominent scientists, then it became the model of how medical education should occur – *and not occur*. This led to the medical licensing laws that we still have today.

This is particularly well-documented in the case of the United States in the 1910s, when the Carnegie Foundation requested prominent physician Abraham Flexner to issue a report detailing what the future of medical education should be in the United States.

When published, Flexner's report was highly critical of medical education for failing to systematically embrace the machine concept of the human body – *and reject other paradigms.*

 Following the publication of his report, educational and governmental licensing reforms were enacted to prevent the operation of any medical school that did not embrace the machine paradigm of human bodies as the exclusive paradigm.

The reasoning was: if the body is like a machine – and the ghost in the machine did not matter – the care of the body should only be entrusted to those who receive "proper" scientific education.

----

[4] For more on the topic of paradigms please see, *The Structure of Scientific Revolutions* by Thomas Kuhn

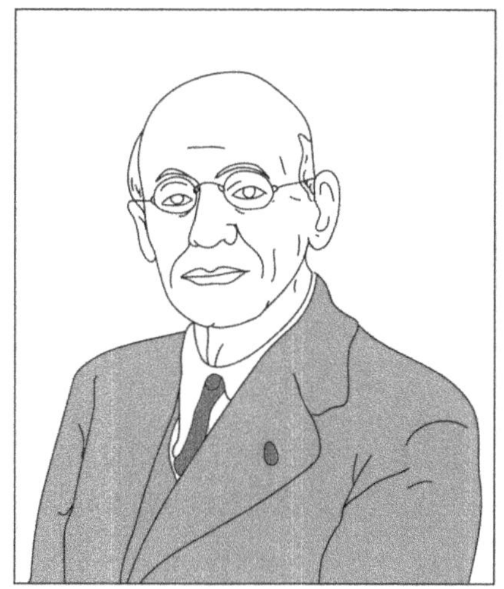

Ever since then, and to this day, medical school entrance requirements have mostly focused on mastery of physical sciences that would fit with the accepted idea of working on a machine.

Even acknowledging there might be a ghost *in* the machine has been discouraged. Flexner influenced a system that ultimately has been antagonistic to anything other than the machine paradigm.

Using the machine paradigm and trying to define health as the "absence of disease" – of a part of the machine not operating at its optimum – makes a lot of sense; the machine model is very useful to address the *parts*.

However, this created a giant problem when medical science tried to define "health" without recognizing that a "Whole Person" even *exists*. This left the very definition of health undefined and a blank spot in Western medicine.

Each person knows better. Each person knows they are more than a machine and more than an assemblage of parts. Because of this, I believe the more accurate definition is, stated again:

Health is when a person's physical and mental conditions allow the pursuit of his or her chosen ends. Disease, then, is the absence of health.[5]

In other words, health is not something that can be measured in a beaker or with a ruler but can only be subjectively defined – by the individual themselves.

This definition shifts the relationship between doctor and patient, where they can become partners in a team. The very idea of Self-Care relies on this partnership.

____

[5] Accad, Ibid

CHAPTER 3

THE MACHINE MODEL PROBLEM NO ROOM FOR SELF-CARE

Have there been negative consequences of adopting the "man-as-machine" definition? Yes, the concept of **you** as being in control of your own health care is highly discouraged.

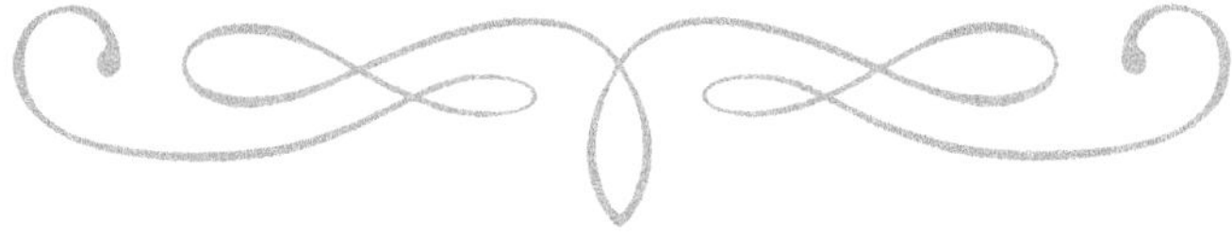

From Dr. Accad,

"If health and disease are viewed as objective conditions to be ascertained by the physician, then the physician is put squarely in control, and patients are passive since their bodies are mere machines." [6]

If our bodies are machines and doctors are the highly trained mechanics, where does Self-Care fit in?

At best, in the back seat. The doctor, the driver, is in the front seat.

This is not an indictment of Western doctors, per se. Many have tirelessly tried to educate their patients to take better care of themselves. And, yes, today more than ever before, there are a large number of online video lectures and resources so that the average person can begin to learn the basics of Self-Care and preventative medicine.

But, even so, the predominant relationship model between doctors and their patients is the "Subject-Expert" relationship where you the patient-subject are being told what to do by the expert-doctor.

This is a far cry from a relationship where you are the "General Contractor" of your health care and your doctor is one of a team of experts you call upon for counsel, advice and services – especially when disease is obviously present.

Consequences of Viewing Disease as the Absence of Health

We define health as being able to pursue our chosen ends. Diseases are conditions that do not allow us to pursue our chosen

[6] Accad, Ibid

ends. Some conditions are obvious and follow common sense: things like heart attacks, pneumonia, and cancer. All of these could conceivably interfere with our chosen ends *permanently.*

But even mild diseases like the common cold can seriously interfere with pursuing our chosen ends. We might have to miss work or a social event because we are down with a cold.

The important consequence of these new definitions of health and disease is that it locates the determination of medical necessity within the patient, rather than in the physician or public health official, since only the patient knows his or her chosen ends – what we may want to do at any given moment.

This also solves the paradox of the healthy blind man; blindness is not automatically classified as a disease if the person can achieve their chosen ends.

From Dr. Accad:

"Under the machine concept of health and disease, a blind person could never claim to be healthy, since a part of the body is obviously and objectively defective. Yet, undoubtedly, many blind persons and many other persons with serious disabilities actually consider themselves to be perfectly well and healthy.

"I believe that they do so because, despite their disabilities and infirmities, they are able to pursue their own chosen ends without undue difficulty." [7]

---

[7] Accad, Ibid

Self-Care as a Partner in Western Health Care

The Western world is in transition and is moving away from the older model of "Subject-Expert" healthcare increasingly toward a "General Contractor" Self-Care model where the individual takes more direct control over their own healthcare.

This does NOT mean that doctors are out of the picture – far from it.

We are changing our relationship to healthcare and our new definition of health puts us in a partnership with those trained in Western medicine.

The patient is the rightful owner of his or her body.

In the course of medical care, he or she delegates control of the body – how much and when – to the physician. The physician is entrusted to work on the body, with the understanding that the goal is to help the patient achieve a condition where they can pursue their chosen ends, to whatever degree possible.

This way of thinking will be new for many people – both patients as well as doctors.

In order for the patient to responsibly either keep control, or delegate control over to a physician, the patient must have some guidelines to go by.

Where do we begin to learn to become the General Contractor of our own health?

CHAPTER 4

HOW TO BECOME THE GENERAL CONTRACTOR OF YOUR HEALTH

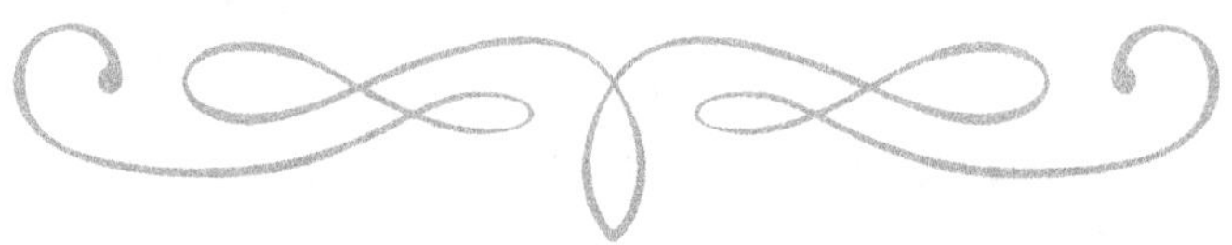

We Westerners are oriented to first look for symptoms and then potential causes.

Although 70% of Americans go for regular medical checkups, both physicians and patients look primarily for obvious complaints and obvious symptoms before taking any action.

In short, we all have been trained to wait until something <u>manifests</u>; something very uncomfortable or even bad is happening before we seek help for it or do something about it. We primarily look at surface symptoms and if we don't see problems, well then, everything is AOK – right?

Our normal reflex is to wait until we "see" or "feel" something and then, say *"Maybe I should get that checked out."*

When should we start to pay attention? How early should we DO something?

The answer is: *as early as possible.* But how do we do that?

We Must Know Where to Begin

Those who embrace the idea of Self-Care could at first feel overwhelmed by the number of options available to them. Today there are countless websites extolling various methods, supplements, therapies and tools. How to choose?

Where does one begin? I know this problem firsthand. When the doctor told me in 2001 to *"Shake hands with your pain"* he followed up by telling me that all he could offer me was a lifetime of pain killers.

That was all he said he could do. Although I said, *"No thank you,"* I did not know where to begin and what to do *first.* I went through quite a long time of trial and error. I was pushed and pulled in several directions by my friends and family that meant well but really did not know more than I did.

I basically had to go back to school. I had always tried to be more fitness conscious but I found that's not necessarily the same as health conscious – or health-educated. I needed to understand how disease starts.

In my case, the neurosurgeon told me that it was genetic, that the facets in my vertebrae had not properly formed in utero. He also told me that he was not sure of that until he actually saw my bones close up. Alternatively, he said, my condition could have been put in motion by either drug or trauma but in my case it was clearly caused by a genetic imbalance.

"Fascinating," I thought, *"so I had a predisposition to it."*

I asked him if my crisis was automatically destined to happen. *"Not necessarily,"* he said.

"So," I thought, *"there must have been some catalyst (or catalysts) that took my imbalance and made it eventually become a crisis."*

I did not realize it then, but at that moment I had recognized what I would later come to appreciate as the first two stages of disease:

- ❖ Imbalance, and
- ❖ Provocation

Choosing to start with what I was most familiar with, I re-embraced fitness and in particular yoga and Pilates. But this time I studied why they worked. During the 1990s I attended yoga classes three times a week for many years. In addition, I gave my employees an hour yoga class every week. But I had never tried to learn why yoga worked.

As time went, on I came to understand that using a variety of different tools and modalities – all focused on regaining balance – was the ticket for me.

Regaining Balance Became My Daily Goal

It started to come into focus. I slept, ate and washed every day to regain balance. My body, I came to appreciate, is wired to regain balance. We rest to feel refreshed. We eat to refuel and feel satisfied. *What we want, the body wants.* And my body wanted to be pain free.

My focus on fitness changed to a focus on regaining balance. At first, I just looked at my daily habits. Then I started to see that I could extend my daily habits into weekly routines. When I finally went back to carefully weight lifting, I saw that my balance was served by three workouts a week.

I started to meet medical professionals who also appreciated the central role of balance and regaining it.

My physician, Dr. James Brooks, M.D., is a remarkable man. Jim has spent a lifetime of study and assisting people regain balance through becoming an expert in several different modalities, including: Psychiatry, Five Element Acupuncture, Zero Balancing and Ayurvedic Medicine.[8]

---

[8] Dr. James Brooks, M.D. is the author of several books, including, *Reflections on Maharishi AyurVeda and Mental Health*, available at http://www.mumpress.com/books/reflections-on-maharishi-ayurveda-and-mental-health.html

I remember asking Jim what the value was of repeating acupuncture sessions regularly. He said, *"Because the body constantly needs to regain balance."*

From that point onward I knew how to select my team of other supporting health experts. Each one would know that balance and regaining it was my goal. It was great if that was their focus – as it was for Jim – but I found that it was more important that I understood this. I could direct my team members to help me constantly regain balance.

As I progressed, I discovered a great term for what I had done. I had become the General Contractor of my Self-Care process.

Meet Your New General Contractor – *You*

A General Contractor, or GC, controls a *process* and is the leader of a team of several contributing members. In the construction of a house, for example, the GC is the primary person responsible and in charge of a project. Let's say that again: *responsible and in charge.*

All of the craftspeople and subcontractors answer to – and are given direction by – the GC. The General Contractor decides which subcontractor to employ at what time and for what part of the project.

The GC knows the *direction* of the project and is constantly making sure that everything's being done to the quality standards required.

The General Contractor must be able to see if he or she is getting what they want from the subcontractors – or not. Sometimes the GC fires and replaces a subcontractor when needed.

Your Project is You

"The Buck Stops Here" was a sign President Harry Truman kept on his desk. It meant that he was the final person in charge. For us, the buck stops with our own health. We are the person ultimately impacted by our own health and the final responsibility rests with us, as our own General Contractor.

However, when it comes to our health we have a choice. We can choose to let imbalance run and let complications advance. We can choose to <u>not</u> be our own GC.

We can ignore early warnings; we can wait for symptoms to manifest and then rush to surrender to a health care provider to tell us what to do to "patch it up." Often times, that patch is too little, too late and, most importantly, may not address the underlying cause.

Or we can step up and embrace our own Self-Care. *If we don't – who will?*

The good news is that we can easily learn to become a General Contractor of our own health and Self-Care.

We can learn how to gain and regain balance.

What To Do First – Learn to Take a Wide Angle View

The following chapter will present a *wide angle view* starting with the most important things I've learned during my own journey. These include:

- ❖ How disease starts and where it comes from
- ❖ How disease grows, manifests, becomes complex and – worst of all – chronic

I'm going to introduce you to a model, a paradigm that will be new to most Westerners and will dramatically increase your control over your own health and Wellness. This model explains how there are six stages of disease – four of which occur BEFORE a disease manifests.

You will understand how disease progresses from imbalance to later becoming manifest, complicated, chronic and even a crisis. Once you know this model you'll own an important tool in *unraveling* the progression of dis-ease and restoring balance for yourself – and largely all by yourself.

This model allows you, the General Contractor of your own health, to more effectively select modalities, tools and lead your Self-Care team. You'll be able to help them work in concert even if some on your team do not understand this model at all.

Once you understand what you can DO to maintain and regain the core element of health – *balance* – you're in a position to become a powerfully effective General Contractor of your own health and Wellness.

CHAPTER 5

THE BIG SECRET: HOW ALL DISEASES BEGIN AND MANIFEST

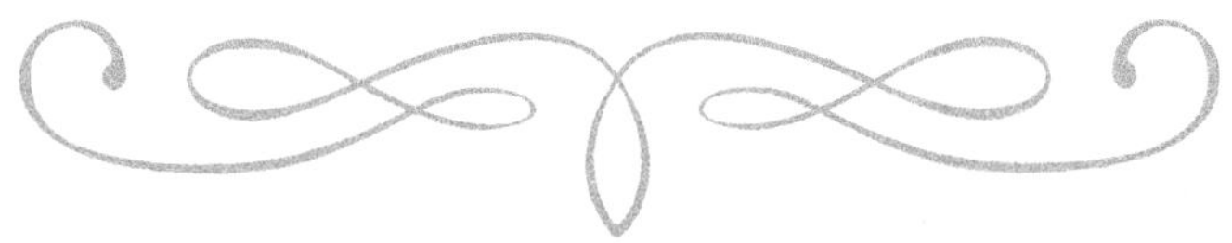

Knowing how disease begins and manifests is the starting point of Self-Care. Ayurveda, the ancient system of health from the Vedic tradition of India, lists six developmental stages of disease:

- ❖ Accumulation of Imbalances and Impurities
- ❖ Provocation (which I like to call Daily Living)
- ❖ Distribution
- ❖ Relocation
- ❖ *Manifestation (when most people start taking action)*
- ❖ Complications, Chronic Problems & Crisis

Disease springs and spreads from imbalances and impurities.

The Problem with Manifestation – It's Often Too Late

Consider the following scenario as presented by Dr. Stuart Rothenberg, M.D., Director of Maharishi Ayurveda Association of America:

"A middle-aged woman complains to her doctor that she just doesn't feel well.She's says she's more tired than usual, a little depressed. The doctor does a physical exam, but doesn't find anything unusual. She also orders blood tests, but these too come back normal. The doctor reassures the patient that she is well, and perhaps encourages her to get more exercise and to come again in six months.

A year later this patient is diagnosed with Type II diabetes.

Unfortunately, this is a common experience in conventional medicine – that the disease cannot be diagnosed until the patient complains of specific symptoms or lab tests demonstrate specific findings.

And by the time the findings are manifest, it's too late to prevent the disease.

The great advantage of the Ayurvedic approach is to identify imbalances before they actually manifest as a disease.

This can allow the Ayurvedic practitioner to take remedial action and reverse the imbalances at an earlier stage of development, thus preventing the emergence of the full-blown disease." [9]

The Role of Prevention

Prevention is the first goal of Ayurveda, exemplified by the old saying, *"Avert the danger that has not yet come."*

More from Dr. Rothenberg,

"Prevention has always been the first and major goal of Ayurveda. Only when the physician has failed in that first goal does he or she need to resort to the second goal – which is cure.

Maharishi Ayurveda identifies six stages in the development of disease. In the first two of the six stages [Accumulation & Provocation], *there are no symptoms. In the third stage* [Distribution] *there may be vague, nonspecific symptoms, such as fatigue and general malaise, which become more pronounced in the fourth stage* [Relocation]. *Only in the fifth stage* [Manifestation] *do symptoms manifest that are specific to a particular disease.*

While conventional medicine uses valuable diagnostic tools to detect disease in an early stage, such as blood tests and X-rays, they are able to detect disease only after it has become physically manifest – for example, a small tumor or elevated blood sugar.

---

[9] The Ayurvedic outline of the Six Stages of Disease is useful for our purposes. For a more complete understanding: http://www.mapi.com/ayurvedic-knowledge/immunity/ayurvedic-understanding-of-disease.html#gsc.tab=0, Accessed Jan 19 2017

According to Maharishi Ayurveda, this would be in the fourth or fifth stage of pathogenesis. Maharishi Ayurveda aims to detect disease at an earlier stage, before it becomes clinically manifest, when the disease process is easier to reverse." [10]

Exploring and Refining the Six Stages of Disease

The Ayurvedic model of disease is very useful in understanding how disease develops and how trauma and pain spreads throughout the body. This model is very valuable in understanding how lower back and other pains manifest.

This outline is not in the detail that can be found in formal Ayurvedic texts. Instead here are a few simple points which are especially applicable to traumas:

- ❖ Manifested ailments have root causes that may be far away from the site of the problem. For example, shoulder or neck problems may have a root cause in your hips, knees or feet, for example
- ❖ You have different levels of control over a disease – either for prevention or treatment – depending on the stage of the disease
- ❖ You, the *General Contractor* of your health, are more effective when you learn to look at these *earlier and at deeper* levels where prevention is possible – the earlier the better

____

[10] Rosenberg, Ibid

Stage One of Disease:
Accumulation of Impurities and Imbalances

Maybe we sit too much, or slouch or don't hold our head up, or round our shoulders. Maybe we were born with a curve in our spine or our diet taxes our liver or our general nutrition is lousy. Maybe we do not drink enough water which makes our tissues overly dry and susceptible to knotting up.

Many of these might be habits that, if we were made aware of them, we might choose to change.

What they have in common is they all weaken us – *unbalance us* – in some way. They set the stage for us to be less resilient and more susceptible to further weaknesses.

The weakness can be chemical. We can accumulate a weaker physiology due to either an overall poor diet or because of one thing in our diet that is especially challenging for our body to process. For some this may be wheat or gluten. For others it may be alcohol or something else.

It can also be the lack of some essential ingredient that we need such as Vitamin D, or it could be – and often is – simply a lack of water.

Whatever it is, it's usually because we are getting too much or too little.

As in most things in life, the right dosage for *you* is the key.

Intelligent choice is the only thing within your power. Paying attention to what works for you – or not – allows you to make that choice. There's only so much we can learn every day and only so much we can know. Take your time; the old saying goes *"you can't eat the elephant all at once."*

Becoming Aware of What is Happening is a *Process*

It's going to take time and you're going to go through changes and adjustments over time.

Therefore, making the more intelligent choice – for you – must become a habit. Self-Care is made up of positive habits we discover, then nurture, and then keep doing.

Some of us were born small, others large. Some tall, some short. All of us have physiologies with various strengths and weaknesses that were built in. Some of these imbalances are more ingrained in our DNA that we may have to contend with over and over for all of our days.

Some imbalances are momentary, and show up simply as a part of living through a normal day.

It's not practical to think we are going to live in the world and not accumulate some impurities or imbalances – every single day. That would be like walking down a hot and dusty road and expecting you won't be dirty and thirsty at the end.

We regularly bathe and brush our teeth precisely because we *accumulate* impurities on a daily basis.

We sleep every night because we *accumulate* fatigue.

A great deal of our personal power and control is recognizing when we are in an imbalanced state and then choosing to do something about it – or not do something, or stop doing something – then and there.

The longer we put off bathing and rest, the dirtier and more tired we will become.

While prevention is important and even ideal, it does not mean sitting in a sterile room and withdrawing from living in the world. Prevention is, rather, not submitting ourselves to obvious problems if we can, and always keeping an eye out to *"avert the danger that has not yet come."*

<u>Stage Two: Provocation</u>

I like to refer to this stage as "Life and Living" because it happens all the time to all of us. Some of these provocations are *Quick & Fast*, some are *Slow & Building* provocations.

Slow & Building Provocations

Like the water level about to burst a dam, little provocations can also accumulate. Think of them as tiny micro-cracks. As more cracks appear and link together with other cracks they accelerate the weakening process. Finally, one teeny crack appears and we finally notice that the dam is leaking.

Like this, we can accumulate an impurity or an imbalance to the point to where we start to notice it.

We've all had this experience.

Every time I

- ❖ *... drink coffee after 3PM ... I sleep poorly.*
- ❖ *... stay up after XX o'clock ... I drag through the next day.*
- ❖ *... don't exercise for a week ...*
- ❖ *... stand too long ...*
- ❖ *... sit too long ...*

The list goes on and on.

Once we cause one of our parts or systems to be overburdened – or overtaxed we provoke bigger problems.

We may not know where and when this bigger problem is going to show up.

Slow & Building provocations are the causes of the future (unpleasant) surprises that await us – later.

Quick & Fast Provocations

Say you missed a stair-step, started to fall, caught yourself, stubbed your toe or slightly hurt your ankle. We could consider this common experience a *Quick & Fast* trauma that has a relatively small short term consequence.

Larger *Quick & Fast* traumas from bad car accidents or falling down on ice have, of course, bigger impacts and longer term consequences.

Provocations can be emotional as well, like unexpected news (good or bad), from winning the lottery to learning of the death or injury of a loved one; these can bring a shock that has real physical effects.

We are constantly dealing with being startled by sudden loud noises or being banged around in one way or another.

Provocations Put All the Later Stages in Motion

We can't stop these random insults from happening. It's not our fault.

Once provocations happen, whether *Quick & Fast* or *Slow & Building*, we are in the regaining balance business. Our job here is to focus on regaining our balance the best we can. This is, of course, our choice. But if we do not, then these provocations move on into the next steps.

Stages 3, 4 & 5: *Distribution, Relocation & Manifestation*

These three stages work together and naturally follow each other.

Let's use the example that you broke your ankle.

This trauma *distributes* the trauma from your ankle upward and may cause you to walk in such a way that puts additional stress on your knees and hips. This in turn changes your spinal alignment whenever you walk, sit and stand.

This ankle trauma may cause a change in how your spine supports your upper back and may, in short order, *relocate* to your shoulders or neck.

Then, later, it can *manifest* as a new pain in the shoulder or neck.

Why is this so? *Because everything is connected to everything else.*

Our fascial and connective tissue matrix is highly interconnected and follows specific physical paths, like "train tracks," that one can easily learn about.[11]

A specially trained bodywork therapist will immediately start looking for other places in the body that could be the cause(s) of a symptom. *Problem in the right shoulder?* They'll look at the left hip as well as down the left leg, and so on.

According to Ayurveda, the progression of the provoked imbalance moves and *"begins to circulate in the body."* [12]

Importantly, in this *distribution stage* there may not be specific symptoms. However, there can be *"vague, low-grade non-specific symptoms, such as transient aches and pains or mild malaise. The patient may complain of fatigue or mild depression or just say 'I just don't feel well.'"* [13]

In the *relocation stage* the imbalance localizes in the tissues of some specific area. This could be like the neck in our example above, or it could be a specific organ. Once the imbalance relocates, it begins to disrupt the functioning of surrounding tissues.

Eventually the imbalance *manifests* as a clear, identifiable problem. The functioning of the tissues or organs are now obviously disrupted. In our example, what started as a problem in our ankle has now developed into a painful shoulder or neck issue. Unfortunately, this is when most people start to seek treatment, when the horse is already out of the barn.

------

[11] Myers, Thomas, *Anatomy Trains*, https://www.anatomytrains.com

[12] Rothenberg, Ibid

[13] Ibid

Disease Stage Six:
Established Complexity, Chronic Problems & Crisis

At this stage the imbalance has manifest and has become so embedded that the body's natural repair mechanisms are not able to reverse it without serious intervention – if it is even possible at all.

At this stage the risk exists of a long-term or even permanent disorder. The longer it goes untreated the more knotty and complex it can become and even develop into a crisis.

We have different action options in Stage Six depending on whether we are experiencing something that is starting to become complex, whether it has become a chronic condition or we are in full blown crisis.

Next we'll examine our action options depending on whether we are in *complexity, chronicity or crisis* which I'll define now.

Complexity and Chronicity

After a problem manifests it can link up with other imbalances which – together – can create a more complex situation. So you can see from this the necessity to *keep the focus on regaining balance.*

Each little imbalance joins hands with other imbalances in such a way that when one imbalance finally manifests others are ready to help make a bad situation worse.

Chronic problems, we could say, come about when a manifested and complex problem takes root. Once a chronic condition sets up shop it can grow to become a crisis over time.

Even when you have a manifested problem, even when it is somewhat complex and even when it is chronic, there are things you can do yourself.

#1 Regain Balance

Fortunately, there are certain things we can do to quickly restore some balance to our system. There is an old analogy from India that in order to stop water from a rolling boil all you need to do is to add a small amount of cold water and the boiling pot will quiet down.

Even a small amount of a balance-restoring strategy may be valuable at this stage. We will explore these more in our chapter on *Building Your Own Tool Kit* in Chapter 9.

#2 You will probably need guidance

Ask for directions! Don't be arrogant and proud. Reach out to others to help you find the right team member to assist you.

#3 Believing + Learning + Action = Let the Unraveling of the Imbalances Begin

You are not helpless and there is more that you can do than you may believe at this moment. Once you *believe* you can heal you have actually started the process of healing.

But you need more than just wishful thinking. Believing, backed up with learning and action puts healing in motion.

Crisis

If you are in crisis don't fool around. Here intervention by a highly trained physician/therapist – and even emergency action – may be required.

The concept of Self-Care includes knowing when you can manage yourself and when you're in over your head. If you find yourself in crisis you must take care of the immediate situation and be responsible for yourself – by asking for help from qualified health professionals.

If you are in crisis you need to take action – NOW – without delay. Above all else, always be responsible for yourself.

The Value of Learning This Model

Even though Ayurveda is a rich and wonderful health care modality, you don't need to seek out an Ayurvedic physician in order to derive great value from the knowledge of this ancient tradition.[14]

Simply knowing these *Six Stages of Disease* provides an orientation, a compass for our health that is very empowering for your Self-Care process. The key action steps from Ayurveda are:

- ❖ Pay Attention – Be aware! There is a lot you can do all by yourself.
- ❖ Stay Balanced – Daily living is going to challenge you.
- ❖ Regain Balance – The body is BUILT for regaining balance.

---

[14] Up until the 1970s Ayurveda was unknown to the Western world. Presently there are several schools of Ayurveda offering products and services. Are they all equal? In my opinion, no. I endorse Maharishi Ayurveda offered by http://www.mapi.com

- ❖ Look Deeper — Make it a habit and discover what works best for you.
- ❖ Know When to Reach Out for Help — Build your Self-Care Team. Self-Care is not Alone-Care.
- ❖ Do No Harm! — Always be responsible for yourself

Next we'll discuss the Four Dance Steps to Wellness.

CHAPTER 6

DESPERATION TO CELEBRATION, FOUR STEPS TO WELLNESS

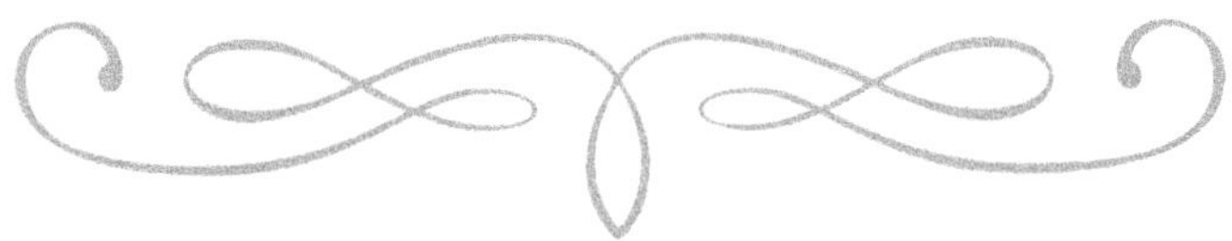

My journey has had many ups and downs, many plateaus and stages. I prefer to think of experiencing Wellness as more like dancing, flowing between four definite steps:

1. **Coping**: Finding Relief and Moving Toward Management

2. **Progress**: Moving Past Management Toward Improvement

3. **Overcoming**: Learning to Get Past Obstacles, Stuck Points & Setbacks

4. **Celebration**: Learning When and How to Celebrate Wellness

Before we discuss each one let's briefly discuss where we want to go, to Wellness.

What is Wellness anyway? How do we create Wellness in our life? Let's recall our definition of health:

Health is when a person's physical and mental conditions allow the pursuit of his or her chosen ends.

Building on our definition of health, we can define Wellness as:

Wellness a state of mind of satisfaction and celebration. We feel Wellness when we can do pretty much everything we want to do and live pretty much the way we want to live.

Why the qualifier *pretty much?* Let's be realistic; our desires are infinite. No matter how good our life is we can always think of a higher ideal.

One day I was sitting at a lunch counter seated next to a guy in his early forties who I'd known only casually. While chatting he said,

"I've recently been experiencing a pain in my back. I've never experienced pain before in my life and I'm having a really hard time with it."

You can imagine my surprise. I said, *"No pain, anywhere, ever?"*

To which he said, *"Yes, nowhere ever. This is a new thing for me."*

Still incredulous, I said, *"Surely you've fallen or been scraped up or something."*

He insisted, *"Nope."*

Upon further questioning it came out that the pain he was now having was, by my observation, pretty mild and not chronic. Most of us who've dealt with chronic pain would simply accept his as relatively small and temporary; more in the 'bothersome" fly-buzzing-about-my-head category. But to him it was a big deal. To him, he was not living *"pretty much the way he wanted to live."* To him, he was not celebrating Wellness.

Defining *Wellness,* like pain, health or happiness is subjective. We will all define it somewhat differently. But what we will all have in common is some feeling of celebrating how great our life is.

Wellness, therefore we will describe as a feeling of satisfaction, momentary or longer lasting, that we alone feel. It is a feeling of ease in the body, mind, heart or soul. And you know it when you're experiencing it.

This is not to say that Wellness is beyond the reach of some people experiencing some advanced stage of some debilitation or disease. Some poor souls face truly insurmountable challenges and unfortunately may not be able to reach it or even taste it.

This may also be true. If that is our reality, perhaps all we can do is give thanks to the few blessings that we can still count even if the number is small.

For most of us there are many action steps we can take that are directly in our power:

- ❖ Even if experts tell us it is impossible
- ❖ Even if the mountain looks way too big
- ❖ Even if we feel completely worn out and, most importantly,
- ❖ Even if we are despairing

Great pain-free health for some, like my friend at the lunch counter, is a gift they don't have to think about. They are simply enjoying their great good fortune and I say, may God continue to bless them for all of their days!

Those of us not so lucky may have to work for our Wellness and health. For some of us not in the state of *acceptable Wellness* could benefit from a road map to help us make it happen. These steps I have outlined may help.

Everyone's steps, path and process to Wellness are different. Actually the steps are more like dance moves that flow back and forth. But before we discuss the dance let's outline the steps and how they can keep you focused on your Wellness goals.

Dance Step #1 is Coping: Finding Relief and Moving toward Management

The scariest part of severe chronic back pain is not knowing how it came about and how to find immediate relief. The first step is relief:

"I want it and I want it right now."

Initially this may mean medications or physical therapy or even surgery. But as many of you know who have consulted with a surgeon for back pain he is going to have you exhaust all lesser invasive options first.

He or she will send you to physical therapy or spinal injections to see if they can help before performing surgery on you. The focus is on *relief:* is there anything that can give you immediate relief or point the way to more sustained relief? Are there any therapy or Self-Care options which can help you to become *well enough?*

I remember when the pain was so great that I had to crawl on my hands and knees into the bathroom to relieve myself. The effort to travel those mere few feet was harder than the hardest rock climb I'd ever done.

At that moment I just wanted to get through that moment! Our total focus is to get through this the best way we can. Here we are at the lowest level of Wellness and all we want is to get out of this terrible situation. Surrendering to our doctor may be our best Wellness strategy here.

In Step 1 you want to get through the moment the best way you can while starting to put together a path to progress. You may be foggy about the details, but you are on your way.

Creating a Team

Within Step #1 we must start to create a team. Our doctor or doctors are key members of our team.

But so are you.

The biggest two things you need to do are: *be on your side and be your own inner coach.* You not only need to tell yourself you can do it, you have to be tough *and* kind to yourself at the same time. This is something many of us were not taught to do. At this point finding out how to listen to yourself is very important for your progress and most importantly for you, as the leader of your Wellness team.

Becoming my own Self-Care Coach
and Listening to my Inner Conversation

Self-care is self-love. Not ego love. Not puffed-up vanity love.

Self-care is deciding: "I'm worth it." Self-care is encouraging yet demanding, patient, kind yet accepting no BS from yourself.

Of all the people in our life there is one who we will be with from our first breath to the last and that is our *self.*

Of all the people we may love in our life, loving ourselves and cultivating a healthy love of our self is essential to obtaining and maintaining Wellness.

It's an old saying, *"If you believe you can or you cannot – you're right!"*

And it's true. What you repeatedly tell yourself is the basic frame – the basic lens – through which you look at life.

My friend, Dr. Charles Coram, author of the great book, *Medical Intimacies,* asked me when I first started seeing him, *"What is it you say to yourself about the challenges and pain that you are facing?"*

I didn't hesitate. I said,

"I tell myself that it's a mistake and shouldn't be there."

For me this was easy. I hold it inside that any pain I am experiencing is not who I am and that it is not my permanent destiny. It is not me and it's not "my pain." I do not own it nor does it define me.

I hold it that there are things I can do to lessen and even eliminate pain. I tell myself that it's my job to find these things and to do them.

And I told Dr. Coram that I tell this to myself almost every day and especially when things get challenging for me. This is my lens and it has served me well. I discovered long ago that the power of my own "self-talk" – both positive and negative – cannot be over-emphasized.

A Quick Exercise

Throughout your life you will come across many people who will tell you to think negatively, to train your inner voice to negatively BELIEVE this or that about yourself, to say to yourself:

- ❖ I can't
- ❖ I'm not
- ❖ I won't
- ❖ I'll never

I recommend you make a list right now of all these negative things you're telling yourself RIGHT NOW. Also, write down what someone's told you in the past, or even today, or something negative you may have told yourself about yourself in the past.

Some *cannots, or won'ts, or nevers,* on your list might have even been true – once long ago – or may, in fact, be *temporarily* true for you today. It doesn't matter.

What matters is that you
LEARN WHAT YOU ARE SAYING TO YOURSELF!

Here is my list of *cannots, won'ts* and *nevers,* I told myself in 2001 right before and right after my spinal fusion surgery:

- ❖ I can't lift my daughter
- ❖ I can't carry something out to the car
- ❖ I can't sleep through the night
- ❖ I can't make breakfast
- ❖ I can't sit
- ❖ I can't stand
- ❖ I can't walk slowly
- ❖ I can't twist even a little
- ❖ I can't exercise like before
- ❖ I can't think straight
- ❖ I can't feel at peace

Or, even worse, I was negative in a very sneaky way, by saying to myself *positively:*

- ❖ I have a sense of losing it
- ❖ I don't have any patience
- ❖ My future is at risk
- ❖ I'm filled with anxiety

All of these say you do not have power to change your condition. You must realize that each of these statements, while perhaps temporarily accurate, are a mistake.

These are all variations on one phrase, *"I don't have a choice."*

This phrase is the biggest poison-pill of all. And the next problem with this statement, *"I don't have a choice,"* is that it's constantly being reinforced in our lives by the media and what we call entertainment.

My wife and I have made it a little game of being the first one to point out when, in a movie or TV show, one character eventually says, *"I don't have a choice!"*

We see several variations of it. Sometimes we'll hear, *"<u>We</u> don't have a choice!"*

Watch for it, you'll be amazed. This phrase pervades our culture. TV shows and movies repeatedly say this – and emphasize this – like no other message. This could be a much larger conversation but let's focus on why this statement *"I don't have a choice"* is so poisonous.

I'm convinced that what you and I tell ourselves *to* ourselves is the most important factor in *shaping* our reality, our future and our Wellness.

Notice I said *shaping.* I did not say creating.

The distinction is that we shape our reality with our thoughts and our inner conversation while we create our reality with our actions.

Loving ourselves and believing in ourself is a key to meaningful and effective action. Practice saying *"I can, I will, I'm going to"* – and it will happen if you back it up with your actions.

Dance Step #1 is first about coping with the situation, finding relief, building a team to support you and about you getting the proper grip around your inner conversation with yourself. Progress may be slow but even a little progress and you're already moving onto Dance Step #2.

Dance Step #2:
Moving Past Management Toward Improvement

You may not see or believe it right now but there are many things you can do and it all starts with believing and planning. Here you start to put a plan in motion, into action.

After my back surgery in 2001 I was unable to stand at the kitchen counter to make a sandwich.

I could walk but could not stand still in a line, like at the grocery store, for more than 30 seconds without sitting down for a few minutes. Doctors diagnosed the ongoing pain in my legs, after several MRIs, to be incurable peripheral neuropathy.

The biting and stinging pain in my legs was so severe that I would lie in bed and visualize my legs were outside of a tent in an ice storm. I could only comfort myself with the thought that at least "inside the tent" the rest of my body was somewhat comfortable and cozy. It was hell.

Goals

Every day I was planning for my improvement and looking for the means to bring it about. I made only two goals. One, I wanted to be able to make a whole meal since I loved to cook and, two, I wanted to be able to take my then-seven-year-old daughter to Disney World in Orlando, Florida. At that moment both of these goals seemed unattainable.

I cried a lot. My wife held me a lot. The doctors, although kind, told me they had done all they could do. So I got busy and a year later we went to Disney World, and today I can make a meal anytime I want (although my wife still pesters me to also clean up the dishes!).

- ❖ Moving to Improvement begins with making goals which includes believing them even if they seem beyond reach today
- ❖ After that comes action, testing and trying things out
- ❖ Next, paying attention to what works and does not work
- ❖ Next, keep up the pace and keep focused on action
- ❖ Next, modify as needed and keep on doing what works

Most likely, things exist that you can do to improve your condition. You only have to:

- ❖ Believe they are there,
- ❖ Keep looking until you find them
- ❖ Do them, and
- ❖ Keep on doing them

Sometimes the hardest part is helping ourselves believe that improvement is possible.

Here being unreasonable can be a good thing. Believe it anyway. You just might be right!

Dance Step #3:
Learning to Get Past Obstacles, Stuck Points & Setbacks

After my 2001 surgery I was told to not engage in serious exercise for 3 months and to do no exercise at all for at least 6 weeks. So in week 7 I made it a point to start with light exercise, or so I thought.

I worked out about 30 minutes most days and after 2 months increased the intensity. One day I did 35 standing squats and I did them as quickly as I could. This was, in retrospect, a big mistake.

To my surprise my left knee literally blew up to be the size of a soccer ball and I had to have the fluid drained off of it and receive a cortisone injection followed by even more recovery time. Then I started all over again.

Setbacks happen. Get up, brush yourself off and start again. It's what I had to do and it's likely what you'll have to do too.

A New Look at the Word *Discipline*

The word discipline has a bad rap. It's directly associated with pain and punishment. *"If you do that you'll be disciplined."* What's the fun in that? Let's look at the word discipline differently.

A *disciple* is one who loves their teacher or what they are learning. When we discipline ourselves we don't have to be harsh. We can frame it that disciplining ourselves is loving our self.

Notice I'm not talking about hurting myself in the name of self-love. Every bit of self-love has to be encouraging and kind-yet-firm.

Perseverance is Willpower + Direction

Perseverance is knowing where you're going and moving toward that goal patiently, deliberately and with as much self-love-discipline needed until you accomplish your goal.

About a year after my 2001 surgery I had tried a 90-day get-fit course that required bicycling and swimming every day. The problem was I hated bicycling and swimming every day. Neither of these activities were my thing. And the funniest thing, I was getting fatter not fitter.

The pain in my legs was lessened by the exercise – so that was good – but I was struggling to maintain the routine. It's very hard to persevere when you dislike what you're doing.

My wife suggested Pilates so I tried it and liked it. From there I moved onto Gyrotonics® which was awesome and started to see real progress – Yay! When I eventually accidentally discovered, of all things, rock climbing, everything started moving even more my way.

It was in the summer of 2002 and we were in Traverse City, Michigan during their Cherry Festival.

One day I stayed at the beach while my wife and then-8 year old daughter went to the festival area without me. When they returned my wife excitedly told me I had to come back with them downtown because our daughter had been awesome on a rock climbing wall. They both wanted to show me and my daughter wanted to do it again – so we all went.

While I stood to the side of the rock wall and held the video camera recording her climbing I noticed her stopped about halfway up the 20+ foot wall. Focusing the camera I could tell she was saying something to herself. After a pause she continued to the top, hit the buzzer and then was lowered down, happy.

Later I asked her what she was saying to herself when she had paused in the middle of her climb.

She said, *"I was telling myself that I could do it."*

Well, for me, it was as if the heavens opened up. It may seem maudlin to say but, for me, hers was an angel's voice I needed to hear. I felt energized and inspired by my little girl's words.

When we returned home I called a lady we knew who volunteered at a local rock climbing gym. I asked her if she thought a middle-aged, overweight guy with health challenges could rock climb.

Thank God she said *"Let's find out!"*

For the better part of the next year on most Saturday mornings we would meet at the gym. She had a daughter the same age as ours and they would rock climb under my friend's supervision. She taught me how to belay and the basics of climbing. I loved it and, thankfully, so did my daughter.

I also learned how rock climbing fulfilled several aspects of my recovery plan and process.

 # 1, it was fun.
 # 2, it required both short-term goals and embracing
  a long-term process.

I found out that it typically takes years to develop really great grip strength and, true enough, it took years of perseverance to go from my skinny T-Rex arms to the Popeye arms and grip I have today.

I learned the safest (and cheapest) way to rock climb is to *boulder* where you're only a few feet or even few inches above the padded floor but you're moving sideways along the wall. I discovered leaning back on the wall dramatically relieved compression in my back, especially my lower back.

A few years later, I ventured out onto real rock and luckily found my rock climbing mentor and great friend, Matthew Fienup in Ventura, California.[15] Matthew and I have since had many great trips together throughout the best climbing areas in California: such classics like Yosemite, Bishop, Joshua Tree and many others. All of these great steps began with an unrelenting desire to discover what would work for me.

It may sound dramatic but I believe that anyone can create their own version of this story for themselves if only they try.

I had discovered a way of having fun and having short term and long term goals that, for me, were fundamental to moving forward. Rock climbing has served me to this day and remains an intrinsic part of my Wellness program.

Rock climbing also inspired me to research ways to become a better rock climber.

In 2003 I met my friend and personal trainer Frederico Gama. I handed him a copy of an awesome book by Brad Johnson titled *"Bodyweight Exercises for Extraordinary Strength."* [16]

I told Fred my plan was to be able to do everything in this book in

---

[15] Matthew's excellent rock climbing school suitable for all age groups, http://www.earthworksclimbing.com/page1.html

[16] Johnson, Brad, *Bodyweight Exercises for Extraordinary Strength,* https://www.amazon.com/Bodyweight-Exercises-Extraordinary-Strength-Johnson/dp/0926888781

three years or less. Here's the interesting punch line. At the end of three years I could do most of the book and something more. I found out what I could do <u>and what I should not do</u>.

I learned that my back surgery created some real boundaries – new boundaries – that I must accept. Most importantly I learned:

- ❖ Much more clearly where these new boundaries existed, and
- ❖ These new boundaries were a lot wider than I imagined – or feared

Accepting what you can't do anymore is part of achieving your Wellness goals.

I was told by the surgeon that I shouldn't try to twist anymore – even a little – due to the cage of metal in my lower back. But what I found out is that I could *modestly* twist, but only so far and only so often and not repetitively. This is what my friend and chiropractor, Dr. Charles Coram, in his book refers to as my "Edges." These are my practical boundaries that are definitely there but are a great deal wider than I had first thought.[17]

In other words, I should not do a Tai Chi twisting exercise where one twists around a hundred times in rapid succession. Also, I found that backbends and jack-knives were a problem that I should avoid. So they become a "maybe later" thing to tackle and frankly, now in 2017, they are still on that maybe list.

So I gave up golf which I liked and found rock climbing which I love.

---

[17] Medical Intimacy, Dr. Charles Coram, https://www.amazon.com/
Medical-Intimacy-Charles-D-Coram/dp/150437522X/ref=sr_1_1?s=books&ie=
UTF8&qid=1490643766&sr=1-1

Some people may read the above sentence and throw away this book, and that would be a shame

I have a friend, we will call Tim, who tells me that if he ever had to quit tennis he would want to die – and he's said it so often that I think he means it. I know of one gentleman who loved to surf in the ocean who, a few months after he decided he shouldn't do it anymore, actually did pass away.

This is sad but telling. This is when your inner conversation can truly be deadly.

If you simply stay open and keep trying you don't know what new adventures are right around the bend and just beyond your current blind spot. Each new adventure is part of your *process.*

Perseverance is a gift. You'll discover new glories along the way. Life will open up. Each new discovery will lead to the next. Your plan will unfold, morph and unfold some more.

Now you see what your plan was in the first place. Your plan is a present you give yourself that continually reveals inner, deeper layers you had no idea were there.

These are gifts you had no idea were inside below the coarse shell of earlier, more desperate moments.

Dance Step #4:
Learning When and How to Celebrate Wellness

These steps of Wellness are more like dance moves we flow between than a stairway that we are climbing. Sometimes it's like allowing some things to fall away, like golf in my case, and embracing new things you never knew were there before, like rock climbing.

Achieving Wellness is a *process.*

We dynamically will need to recommit, refocus and cope – again and again. Some days will be more challenging than others and the habits of patience, perseverance, discipline (the loving yourself kind of discipline) and self-encouragement will always need to be there.

Celebrations will come and they'll be big and small.

- ❖ Take pictures of them
- ❖ Post them on Facebook
- ❖ Send your celebrations to your friends and family
- ❖ Yell out loud all by yourself
- ❖ Jump up and down
- ❖ Write an article about it
- ❖ Start a blog

What will happen is that you'll encourage others, some you may never meet. And just like that, your process helps others with their process.

When you celebrate it uplifts you and so many others.

It's not about calling attention to yourself in the *"Ain't I great?"* kind of way. It's about showing your progress to the world and being grateful for it.

Sometimes, maybe even most times, while all alone you may choose to simply sit, stand, walk, or lay and feel grateful to the Almighty in whatever name you like to call Him or Her.

Hey, that's great too.

DO IT & SHARE IT

Whatever way you want to celebrate your progress is great – do it! And I strongly encourage you to also share it. The person who benefits most is you in oh-so-many ways. Celebrating will assist you to grow in many ways, including:

Perspective

Celebrating a new high point will remind you of your progress and make you value the habits you've cultivated and actions you have taken to achieve that progress.

Gratitude

Celebrating gives you a chance to take a breath and be reminded – and be grateful for – the fabulous team you put together for yourself and the progress you've already made.

Resourcefulness

Celebrating improves your ability to look for and find new refinements and new solutions. BE OPEN!

For every new piece of your tool kit you figure out you are more likely to believe in yourself more, discover even more new tools and be more likely to figure out other challenges.

You begin to think in a new and powerful way. Your go-to inner conversation becomes:

- ❖ What else can I do?
- ❖ What else can I learn?
- ❖ How can I become even better?

Optimism

Celebrating the high points – one moment at a time – helps you get through the lower points, relapses, setbacks and new frustrations that can come along. This is *crucial.*

My surgery was in 2001, and for 13 years I made steady progress. In 2014, I had a serious setback. After hitting a deer with my car I had a "new" bulging disc that was seriously impinging on a nerve and was so painful I was scheduled for another surgery.

But I had come too far to give up my ingrained habits. I tried all the things I had learned but none of them was working for me well enough.

It was then, while lying on an early version of our Gravity Pal® low angle inversion table I felt a shift in my back and knew that something important had happened.

I called my surgeon and we put off that surgery, first for two weeks, and then another two weeks and then we kept putting it off until the surgeon told me, *"Just call me when you think you need it."* That was years ago and I haven't had to have that surgery.

And that was when this book started and that was when I knew I had to continue to develop and share Gravity Pal® with the world.

Celebrating can take two seconds alone in the car merely smiling and saying out loud – ***"Thank you!"***
Celebrate your progress and your wins. *Love your Wellness process.*

CHAPTER 7

CAN INVERSION BE A CENTRAL WELLNESS & SELF-CARE TOOL?

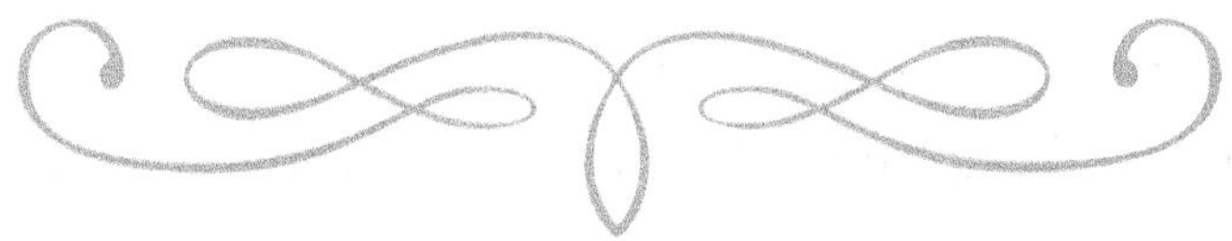

Because back pain is so ubiquitous, using inversion tables is commonly presented as a viable Self-Care treatment and, as part of a healthy lifestyle, it can be.

But when is inversion appropriate? And is it appropriate for everyone?

Let's first address an obvious problem: the public – even the Mayo Clinic at this moment in history – equate inversion with *high angle inversion – only.*

But is high angle inversion the only option? How did we all come to assume it was?

Let's Not Equate the Inversion Table Commercials We See on TV with Self-Care

We see the infomercials on television; fit men and women presenting high angle inversion tables and a parade of buff fitness enthusiasts declaring the benefits they've received from going upside down, and even exercising upside down.

I believe these people are not exaggerating their claims of benefit. But what is wrong with this picture?

What are the differences between these people and the Mom & Pop home audience on the other side of the screen they are trying to sell their products to?

Answer: A Lot.

How did the high angle trend begin and what is it missing? What are the legitimate pros and cons of high angle inversion?

What happens when we look at inversion more broadly, when we go beyond the obvious focus on back pain relief and explore its potential application toward general Wellness?

I believe inversion is one of many Self-Care tools but it can be a *central* tool. Inversion needs to be applied differently for different people. Most importantly, there are multiple considerations and the height of the angle is just one of them.

What about inversion as a central Wellness tool?

Exploring this question is new ground for many people. Currently this is not part of the public discussion.

So let's briefly explore the history of inversion, spend some time looking at high angle inversion as an option and end with summarizing what responsible inversion Self-Care and using inversion as a Wellness tool would look like.

High Angle Tables – The Only Option Since the 1980s

High angle inversion is what automatically comes to mind when most people today think of inversion.

Prior to 1980 those who knew about inversion called it "slanting" which today we would call low angle inversion. Our Gravity Pal® Low Angle Inversion tables are a refinement of this older idea called "slanting."

Nowadays, due to 35 years of television infomercials, low angle slanting options other than Gravity Pal® are non-existent because only higher angle tables are mass-produced.

You may remember if you're old enough, in 1980, when the actor Richard Gere made Gravity Boots famous in the movie *American Gigolo.* Most people do not realize that movie kick started a movement away from low angle inversion and toward radical upside-down and high angle inversion.

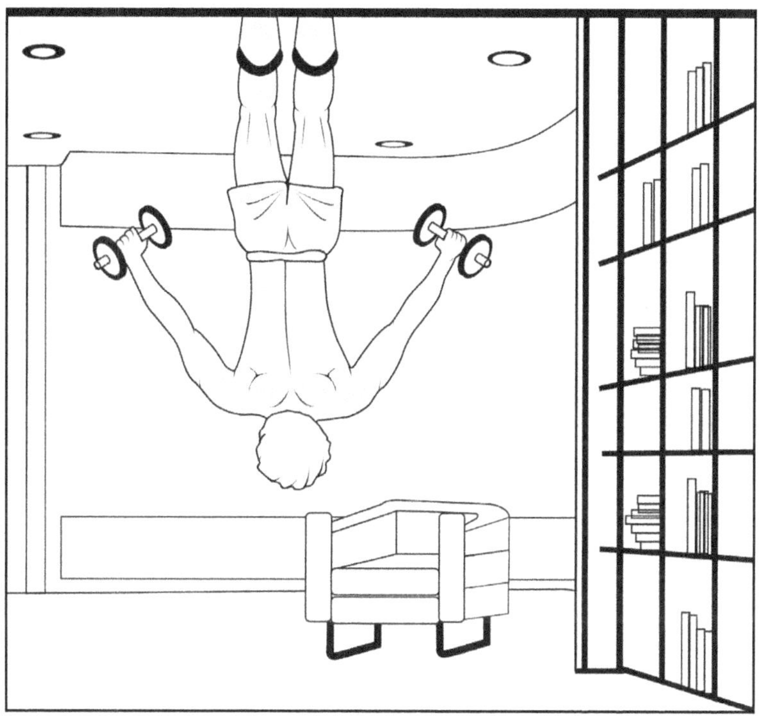

Is Inversion Only for the Very Fittest or Elite Athletes?

Watching late-night infomercials one might be tempted to think so. And, there is a place for higher angle inversion options. Higher angles may be appropriate for elite athletes and those having superior fitness, such as those in military service or those whose professions or hobbies require higher orders of fitness like firemen, mountain rescue workers, gymnasts or rock climbers, for example. And higher angle inversion may be tolerable for certain younger age groups who may be more fit than those who may be older and less fit.

However, high angle inversion may not be appropriate for many people and may be downright dangerous for some people.

Once people get beyond a "certain age" (above 40) they need to be more concerned and conservative about ankle pain, their ligaments being stretched out too far and their internal fluid pressure accelerating too quickly if they go upside down.

Also, high angles, especially when completely upside down, require a spotter just in case the person blacks out or cannot get out of the upside down position by themselves.

What about the rest of us who cannot or do not want to go upside down? What about those of us of modest or marginal health and fitness or those of us who are older?

What about those of us who live alone and don't have a spotter?

Are we just out of luck?
Is inversion simply not available to us at all?

Clearly, high angle inversion has many advocates and happy users. I am delighted these people have discovered the advantages of inversion in general. However, it's a tragedy that a far larger population has avoided inversion simply because they may think – and rightly so – the high angle approach is not a responsible thing for them to try. Many do not know about a viable low angle option.

I am an advocate of responsible inversion Self-Care. Although high angle approaches may be suitable for many people, I believe that lower angle inversion at regular, short intervals is potentially valuable – and more responsible – for a great many people.

But low angle inversion is not simply taking a board and stapling old carpet to it and leaning it up against a couch. Lying on such a thing for 15 or 20 minutes may in fact create new pressure points on the spine and more problems for a person than they were trying to solve.

Similarly, while yoga shoulder stands and yoga headstands may be tolerable and even valuable to some people, they may be very dangerous for other people.

Where is the *sweet spot* where people can approach inversion in the first place? How can they experience it responsibly for themselves?

First let's look at how this problem of finding this sweet spot came about.

A Brief Historical Perspective

The history of seeking relief from gravity goes back to ancient times. There are reports from around 400 B.C. of Hippocrates observing people being tied to ladders, then hung upside down, presumably the patients were volunteers.

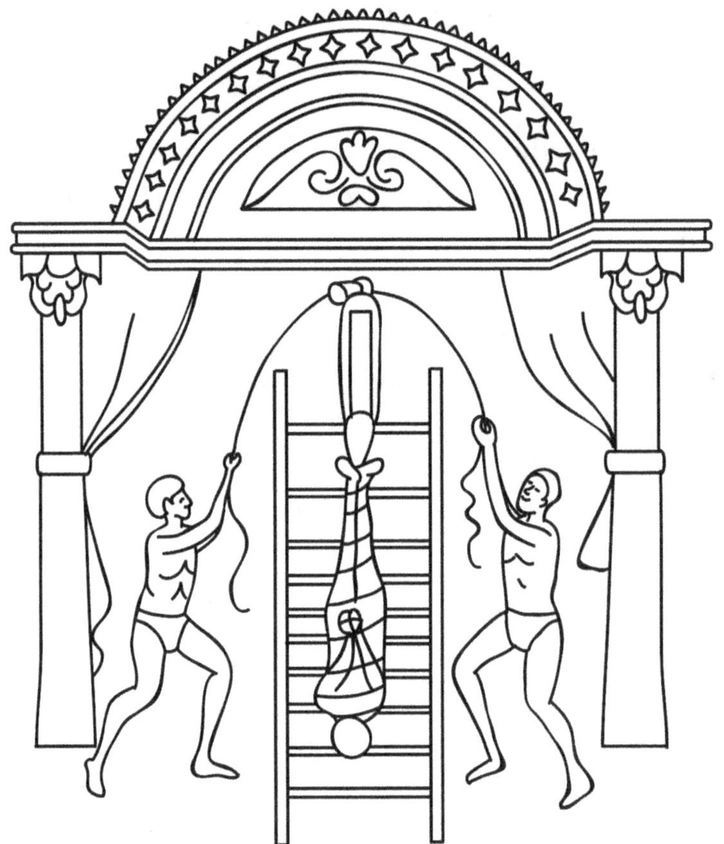

Similarly, if you review ancient yoga texts you find records of various recommended inversion postures from the Shoulder Stand *(Sarvang-Asana)* to Standing on your Head *(Sirsha-Asana)*.

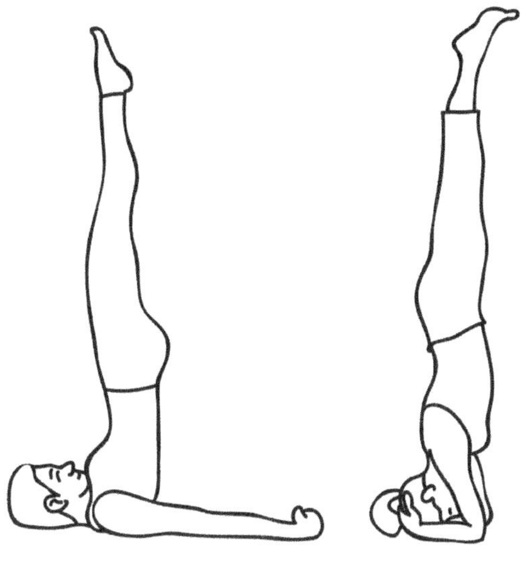

There are similar accounts from the European Middle Ages where they used a system called the *Scamnum (bench of) Hippocrates* which was a ladder-like device used to facilitate inverted traction.

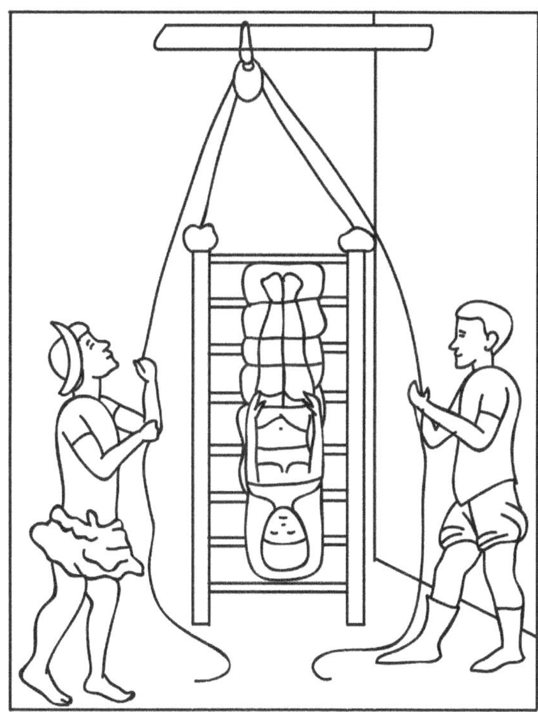

Fast forward to the early part of the 1900s and you start to find numerous patented products that were supposedly going to help one escape the compressive effects of gravity. Some doctors became locally or regionally famous for advocating low angle slanting along with their other programs of diet or Self-Care.

There have been a fair number of interesting inventions along the way which tried to make low angle inversion more convenient but were hard to lie on and were very uncomfortable. Many of these were made for what appears to be smaller people, and mostly women who weighed under 150 pounds.

One such attempt included a 1961 invention which converted a non-padded ironing board into a slanting board *(ouch)*.

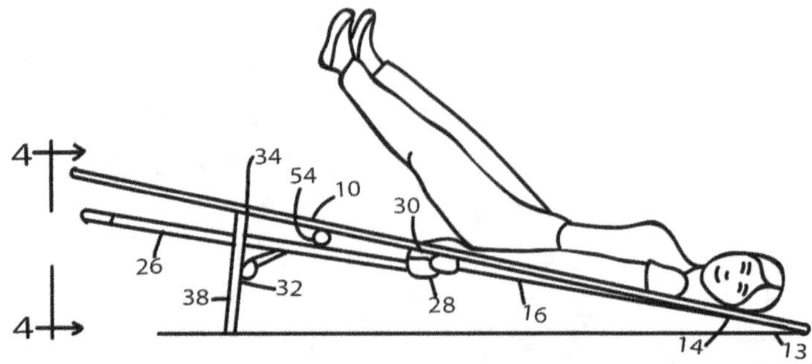

Along the way there were attempts to merge the idea of low angle inversion with exercising.

One emphasized what we today recognize as yoga postures, but in a slanted position. These units were so hard and made of such smooth material that only a very small person who wore sticky clothing could stay on one without slipping off.

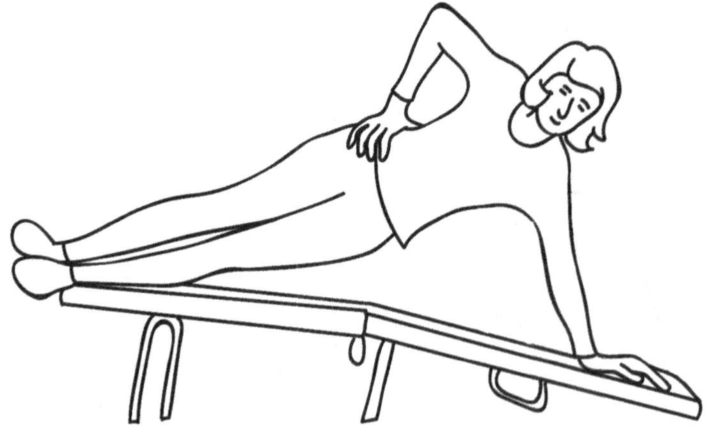

These early devices also appeared in the movies. There is a scene in the 1973 movie *The Last of Sheila* with James Mason, James Coburn and Raquel Welch where, very briefly, you can see one being brought aboard a yacht and being set up for one of the actor's use.

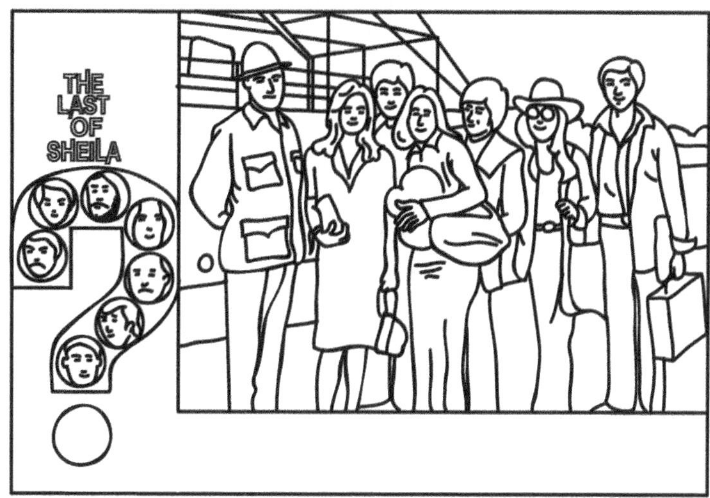

There were many who loved and advocated low angle slanting because, for them it felt good. But this was not a huge trend largely because these lower angle tables, for most people, were quite uncomfortable to lie on.

The Era of High Angle Inversion Begins with Confrontational Exercise

The early era of low angle inversion veered off into radically upside-down high angle inversion largely because of Dr. Robert M. Martin, M.D., an Orthopedic Physician and Surgeon from Pasadena, California who wrote the book *The Gravity Guiding System* in 1975 promoting his own Gravity Boot product.

Dr. Martin also taught gymnastics as a hobby and was personally committed to fitness and health. He referred to his approach as **confrontational exercise** and asked the question, *"Why does* *confrontation exercise work better than operations and medications in many instances?"*

He believed that using gymnastics, which included radical upside down inversion using his Gravity Boots, resulted in a *"veritable fountain of youth for all ages of suffering humanity."*

His comments are not to be quickly dismissed or taken lightly. He was a well-regarded physician who enthusiastically claimed positive results for many people. However, a person had to commit to a very serious regimen of exercise and you had to achieve an advanced state of fitness in order to even get started with his high angle inversion approach.

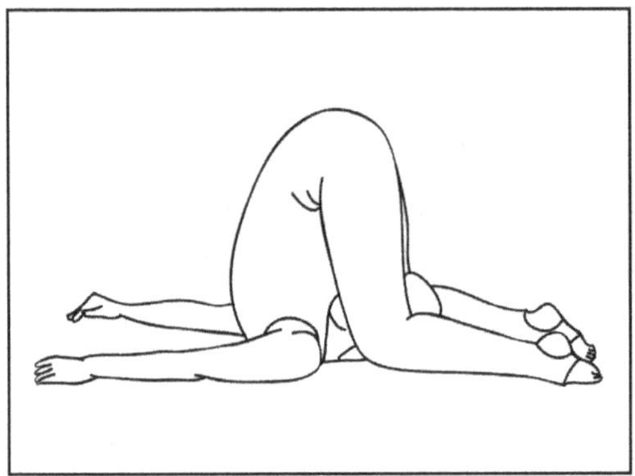
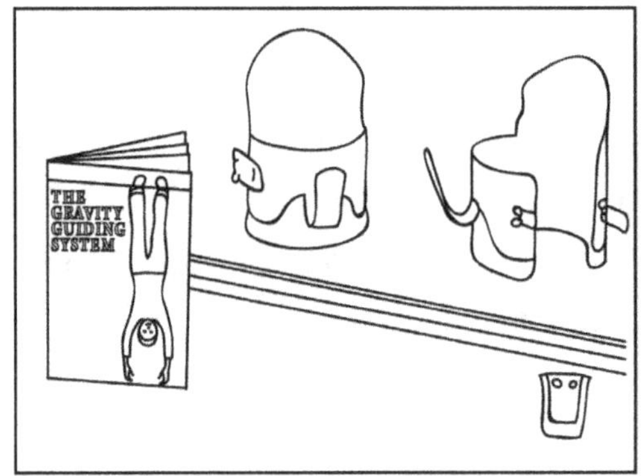

This, for many people of average, modest or marginal fitness, rendered his approach impractical and out of reach. Martin's Gravity Boots looked like a pair of heavy ski boots that had large, strong metal hooks on the front of the boot. A person using these boots had to:

- ❖ Be able to do a full body chin up
- ❖ Once pulled up they needed to rotate their entire body upside down
- ❖ Once upside down they had to pull their legs up over the chin up bar and hook the front of these big, heavy boots on the chin up bar
- ❖ They would then let go and "relax" upside down

Then the Real Fun Began

Once upside down people immediately encountered two BIG issues:

1. A powerful flow of blood would rush to their heads, and

2. Unless they had a spotter they had to <u>all by themselves</u> get right side up again – otherwise they could be stuck upside down.

This, if done alone, was a very dangerous situation.

Those who were less physically fit were left out and had to work up to a specific fitness level before they could invert. They were required to commit to a serious exercise regimen that might take months to complete before they could even try his inversion approach.

Nevertheless, Gravity Boots were made "cool" by Richard Gere's movie performance and they captured the attention of a population that had recently embraced the Jane Fonda Workout and other intense physical fitness workouts in general.

I was unable to find any records showing how Dr. Martin's clients responded to his confrontational therapeutic approach. But he obviously inspired a lot of people, particularly younger people, to try out his Gravity Boots.

My 1982 Experience with Gravity Boots

I remember in 1982 when my friend John proudly showed me his new Gravity Boots.

John and I were both about 31 years old and casually played tennis every so often. One day, while over at his house and he showed me these new boots and what looked like a chin-up bar he'd put up on a door frame. He eagerly urged me to try it out.

John described how to get up on it. I remember looking at it and thinking *"this will be easy."* Ha!

It reminded me of being in the 5th grade and playing on the monkey bars in the school playground. Well, I was in for a surprise!

He helped me put on the too-tight boots. They had these giant hooks on the front.

"It's simple", he said, *"Just jump up, hook your feet on the bar, let go and go upside down."*

What happened next would guide my shoulder therapy for the next 20 years.

I grabbed the bars at shoulder-width and did indeed go *almost* upside down, remembering what it was like playing on the SunnyView Elementary School playground in Mount Clemens, Michigan.

But alas, I was not in the 5th grade anymore!

And I was no longer a crew cut kid who bicycled at least an hour a day delivering newspapers enjoying the blush of young perfect health.

No, I was 31 and not paying attention to the extra pounds around my waist. Nor was I connected with my new lack of bicep/tricep strength. It seems that the previous 10 years of office work and corporate meetings did not yield the same results as exercising on the monkey bars every day when I was ten years old.

So here I go upside down, my feet amazingly coming up almost to the bar and my new fatter belly blocking these heavy boots passage to make any further progress.

"Uh oh," I thought.

Now I was almost upside down, precariously backwards and losing my grip! Thank God my friend came to my aid.

John, my spotter, had witnessed the whole thing. He immediately saved me by lifting my now rounded and inverted body.

He grabbed the Gravity Boots and hooked them over the bar. *"Thank God!",* or so I thought!

At least I was not going to crash below, fall on my neck and most probably break it. I let go and hung upside down. I let out a sigh of relief.

Well, that relief lasted all of about 1.5 seconds. Then came the realization this was not a good place to be and I now had to get off of it and *fast.* I thought my head was going to explode!

Gratefully my red face was very obvious and my full throated *"HELP"* was met with the competent hands and strength of my friend John.

He curled me up, unwound me from my upside down hell and unhooked my feet.

As I stood upright the immediate swirling, nauseous dizziness made me sit right back down.

Total time from start to finish: about 12 traumatic seconds.
I never tried it again.

Funnily enough, I would again pursue gymnastics in another form, rock climbing, many years later.

But going upside down held a special respect. I experienced very clearly that unless:

- ❖ I had a spotter and
- ❖ I was in supremely good shape,

I was *never* going to do that again.

Higher angle inversion was not for me. Maybe it was great for others, but not for me.

Ketchup Bottles, Yoga Headstands & High Angle Inversion Lovers

My friend Tim loves doing yoga headstands called *Shirsh-Asana*. This is when the body, while completely upside down is supported by the forearms, while the top of the head rests on the floor.

Tim told me he's been doing *Shirsh-Asana* every day for 40 years and loves this ancient form of inversion developed in India thousands of years ago.

Tim looks great you'd never believe he's 60 years old. He could easily pass for early 40s and is quick to say that *Shirsh-Asana* is not for everyone; it takes years of practice just to be able to do it correctly (during which time injuries can occur) and even now he sometimes has neck compression problems.

But he loves it and does it religiously about 15 minutes every day – so he tells me.

Tim is among the very few I've ever known who've trained their bodies to be able to fully invert without – so far – creating serious problems for themselves.

For a large percentage of the population radically high angle inversion may not be appropriate and, in fact, may be dangerous.

Yet some people really love and tolerate high angle inversion. To those, I say God bless you. For me it's too scary, there's too much brain pressure and it's definitely not relaxing!

And it's too sudden, too much like being in an upside down ketchup bottle.

To their credit, the manufacturers of high angle inversion tables recommend to always start at a lower angle. But here are three problems about their recommendation.

1. The lower angle they normally recommend is 20 to 30 degrees. This is still a very high angle. By contrast we build our Gravity Pal®at a low angle of approximately 13 degrees.

2. They recommend "working up to" tolerating 60 degrees. Sixty degrees is a *really* high angle!

3. They completely ignore the reality of Muscle Guarding, which is when we tighten up due to our body's natural reaction to pain, instability and/or surprise.

Here's a question:

What happens to the contents of an old style ketchup bottle when you quickly turn it upside down?

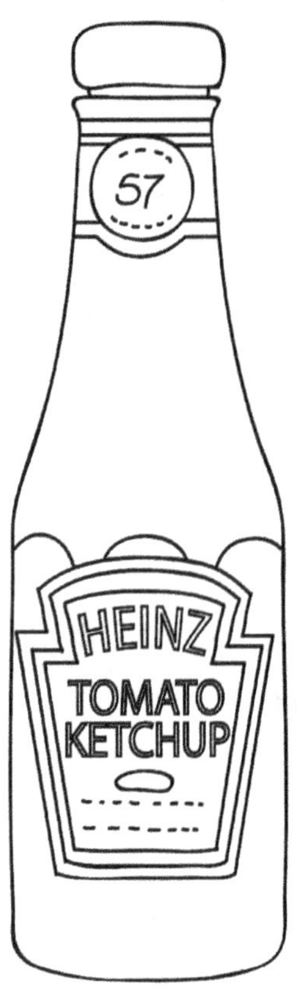

Answer:

The sudden turning upside down <u>stops</u> the flow of the ketchup; it does not promote the flow. Gravity has to "catch up" (pun intended).

Growing up with such old style ketchup bottles, it was most common to smack the upside down bottle hard to try to force out the ketchup. *Great, let's use more force!*

Maybe this is why – finally after a hundred years – ketchup manufacturers are moving away from the old thin necked bottles and to the easy squeeze bottles of today.

Apparently they finally accepted that most people don't want to work so hard to get their ketchup out of the bottle. People would rather work *with* the laws of physics than fight them.

Responsible inversion Self-Care asks:

- ❖ Why work so hard?
- ❖ Why not get immediate results?
- ❖ Why "work up to" a 60 degree tolerance level, risking ankle pain, stretched ligaments or worse?
- ❖ Why not instead use a low angle inversion option that works WITH nature?
- ❖ *Why not do less and accomplish more?*

Other problems with High Angle Inversion

Today, if you Google the words "inversion therapy" you'll immediately come across a post from the Mayo Clinic authored by Dr. Edward R. Laskowski.

Dr. Edward R. Laskowski, M.D. is co-director of the Mayo Clinic Sports Medicine Center and a professor at the Mayo Clinic's College of Medicine.

He ignores the idea of low angle inversion altogether and even defines inversion therapy as *"hanging upside down."*

Dr. Laskowski then states that doing so is *"not safe [and] could be risky for anyone with high blood pressure, heart disease or glaucoma.*

Your blood pressure increases when you remain inverted for more than a couple of minutes and the pressure within your eyeballs jumps dramatically." [18]

---

[18] http://www.mayoclinic.org/diseases-conditions/back-pain/expert-answers/
inversion-therapy/faq-20057951

But there are other problems with going upside down. If you read the user's manuals written by the manufacturers of high angle inversion tables you don't have to read too far between the lines to see that you have to take precautions:

1. To not create ankle pain, and

2. That you should always have a spotter in case you get stuck at an angle that is too high for you

What they do not tell you is that many physicians warn people, especially over 40, to be careful with high angle inversion tables because of the danger of stretching out the ligaments – a really bad thing to have happen.

In other words, the concept of also using a lower angle inversion, for many a more responsible inversion approach, is not even considered.

Beyond the angle issue there are other considerations that are also rarely discussed, like aggravating pressure points, common with many homemade approaches. We will further address this issue in Chapter 8.

What Responsible Inversion Self-Care Looks Like

We've come a long way since the time of Hippocrates when they tied people to ladders. But unfortunately the dominant view of "inversion" as a tool primarily sees at it as a tool for compression relief and only with high angle tables as the available choice.

But that is changing; people are starting to look beyond the obvious and discovering different reasons to use inversion in their lives.

Multiple Uses

Inversion can be viewed as a Self-Care tool for compression relief or as a central Wellness tool – or both. It can be used for a wide range of conditions that have nothing to do with back pain.

An 82 year old lady in very good health told me she maintains a schedule of two daily sessions of a few minutes each time on her low angle inversion table to keep her facial skin looking younger. She swears by it.

Sixty-seven year old Patrick from Pennsylvania uses his Gravity Pal® daily because he says it improves the clarity of his thinking.

A 57 year old broker told me he gets on his low angle table, which he keeps in his office, most days at 3 PM because of the energy boost 5 minutes on it gives him. He calls it his "de-stresser" that allows him to enjoy the rest of his day and evening without being as tired as he used to be.

14 year old Nicki, a high school student, uses her mom's Gravity Pal® to recover from her vigorous dance class rehearsals. Her mom told us this developed spontaneously. Nicki tried it out after one particularly exhausting day and then it simply became routine – she would get on their Gravity Pal® first thing after she got home.

These are all examples of using inversion – not for compression or pain relief reasons but primarily as a Wellness tool. None of these people have chronic back problems but have seen in their own experience the broader value regular, short duration, low angle inversion sessions can bring to their health.

Basic Requirements

Responsible inversion Self-Care starts by taking into account:

- ❖ Age
- ❖ General health condition, and
- ❖ Approximate fitness level of the individual

These three need to be addressed first before someone choses to invert.

Age

After the age of 40 or so, and depending on the lifestyle and fitness of the individual, many people should be aware that the ligaments in the body may not be as strong as they once were. Because of this it may be advisable for them to not use high angle inversion options that could potentially stretch out their ligaments.

What is the upper limit of age? I really don't know. I met a 95 year old lady who not only enjoys her short sessions on a Gravity Pal® but did a backflip getting off of it! We told her we wouldn't advise that for anyone to do, but for her it's no problem.

General Health Condition

While it's advisable for everyone to consult with their physician before engaging in inversion, or any new exercise regimen, it is essential for anyone who is in marginal or poor health to first consult with their primary health care provider.

Some conditions, like pregnancy, clearly disqualify someone from inverting. Others may be okay if a doctor says it's okay to try it.

Whether someone with a particular condition should invert may be directly tied to whether they are thinking of trying a high angle or a low angle option. Again, this should be discussed with their physician.

Approximate Fitness Level

For higher angle options, especially, people should consult their physician. The stresses of high angle inversion must be discussed particularly for people who have any issues in their joints. But even for those considering low angle inversion on a Gravity Pal®, we err on the side of caution and still recommend everyone first consult their physician.

One potential disqualification is for anyone who has difficulty standing up after lying down on a floor. In this case we would recommend the person first build up their strength before attempting even low angle inversion.

Alternatively, if the person could have a readily available assistant to help them get up off of the floor that might be okay. But this is a case that should be discussed with a doctor before considering any kind of inversion, including at low angles.

Inversion is a Powerful Tool which Should be Applied Appropriately

Responsible inversion needs to be appropriately and differently applied for the infirm, the non-athletic, and those in marginal health as well as the elite athlete.

We know of a wife who initially assisted her infirm husband to get on and off their low angle Gravity Pal® so he could invert. It was quite a process. She put up small blocks, like little stair steps that allowed him to get to his knees after inverting and then, with her help, get up to a nearby chair. Even though he would only be on the Gravity Pal® for 1 to 3 minutes, it would take more time for him to get from being on the floor to sitting in the chair.

This lasted for a few weeks before he was able to get on and off by himself. He got stronger. In his case, the severe lymphedema (swelling) in his lower legs started to go down. He had been housebound for several months. Imagine my surprise when, about a month after they started working with the Gravity Pal®, I saw him at a local movie theater!

This is an exceptionally severe example but it illustrates that special care may sometimes be required.

Dosage, Dosage, Dosage

Once it is determined that inversion may be appropriate, the following ***dosage requirements*** need to be addressed:

- ❖ Duration – how many minutes should a session last?
- ❖ Frequency – how many sessions per day?
- ❖ Regularity – When to fit it in? First thing in the morning, or just before bed, or both? Right after work or exercise?

Self-Care involves discovering what you need to give yourself to attain your objectives. The answers to the above questions will be different for different people depending on why they are inverting.

Our experience indicates that all of the above-mentioned elements must be taken into consideration in obtaining the best short-term and *cumulative* long-term results.

We advise Gravity Pal® users follow our *Gravity Pal Inversion Method™* which suggests short durations of 1 to 3 minutes of low angle inversion that are regularly experienced. In the next chapter we will discuss these dosage factors in greater detail.

Only One Tool

Keep in mind that responsible inversion is only one Self-Care tool to consider when you build your personal Self-Care tool kit.

Inversion is only one part of a larger focus on positive Self-Care for Wellness. However, just like brushing one's teeth, responsible inversion can easily become a self-reinforcing daily habit that supports other positive Self-Care practices and habits.

How Do We Create Self-Reinforcing Habits?

Quite simply by making it both convenient and something that people look forward to doing by themselves.

1. Must Be Convenient

Convenience comes in two forms: readily available and easily fitting into our schedule.

Responsible inversion should be available to us whenever we want or need it. We should receive value from it if we have only a single minute available and then continue with our day.

2. Must Look Forward To It

We look forward to something when we get what we want from it.

Once the habit is established we look forward to our inversion sessions and miss them when they're not available for some reason.

The road to Wellness is paved with good Self-Care habits that are easy for us to keep doing.

This includes responsible inversion sessions. Self-care should be easy and something we want to do because we are getting what we want out of it.

Why Isn't Inversion More Universally Used?

Why don't more doctors take inversion more seriously and prescribe it for its potential Wellness benefits beyond its potential for back pain relief?

I think this is about to change as the focus shifts from the angle as the primary issue – to the *combination* of the most responsible angle for the individual and the method used. Both angle and method must be evaluated together.

The first rule of being a healthcare provider is to *do no harm.* The first rule of Self-Care is to do no harm and to approach one's care responsibly.

In the next chapter I'll discuss Gravity Pal® low angle inversion tables in combination with our *Gravity Pal Inversion Method*™ and how they both contribute to responsible inversion Self-Care.

CHAPTER 8

THE METHOD MATTERS: HOW I MADE INVERSION WORK BETTER FOR ME AND MY CLIENTS

Challenges in Developing Gravity Pal®

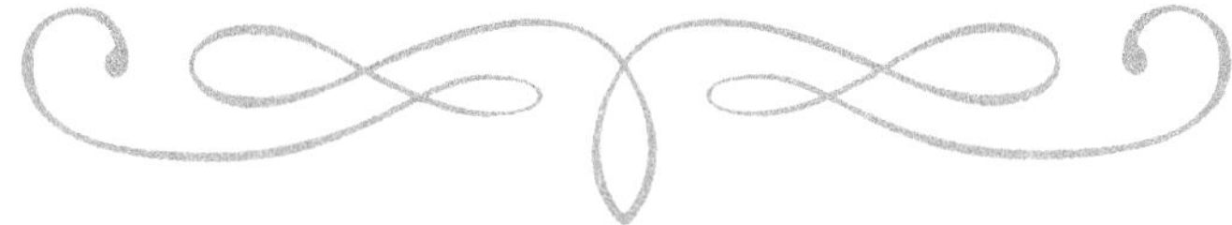

Even though the idea of inversion as a way to escape gravity's effects is quite old, there has, until recently, been no systematic attempt to develop a means whereby the majority of the population, whether young, old, fit or not can accomplish this escape – *and stay motivated to do so.*

There may be several reasons for this, but the biggest, in my opinion, is that the idea of inversion suffers from what I would call being *too obvious.*

Maybe this is why inversion tables have been a late-night TV "impulse buy." And maybe this is one of the reasons so many people have told us they had previously purchased a high angle inversion table that they never use!

They originally thought it was going to give them what they wanted but, somehow, it wound up in their garage or basement collecting dust.

We wanted to develop something that people would use and look forward to using and miss when they could not use it because the daily experience was so positive for them.

Appearing too Obvious and Finding Out It's Not!

Here's a fun story.

My friend Pat is a very fit and friendly guy in his later 60s who uses his Gravity Pal® a few minutes every day because he says it improves his mental clarity.

Pat had mentioned it to his neighbor, Doug, who had been having back issues. He came over, tried it and liked it so much that he came by Pat's house almost every day to use it.

One day Pat announced he was going on a two week trip. Doug asked if he could borrow Pat's Gravity Pal® while he was gone, to which Pat agreed.

When Pat returned two weeks later Doug jokingly told Pat that he didn't want to give back the Gravity Pal® because it was really helping his back.

At this point, Pat asked Doug if he would like to talk to me and that is how I found myself talking to Doug on the telephone one Saturday afternoon.

It was all very cordial with Doug telling me how much the sessions were helping him and how much he appreciated the engineering that went into it. But then, when I asked him if he would like to purchase one he laughed and said, *"Oh no, I could make one of those in my garage in an afternoon. There is no way I would purchase one."*

I told him that I once, naively, had thought the same thing; it would be very simple, quick and inexpensive to make – but after I got into it found out quite the opposite. It was not simple, nor quick, nor inexpensive.

Nevertheless, Doug said that he would certainly be able to figure it out. And, unfortunately, as of the date of this writing, according to Pat, he's never even tried to make one.

We've witnessed versions of this several times. They say this because it looks so obviously intuitive; what more do you have to do? All that is needed is to invert and that should bring compressive relief – *right?*

One of our early customers, Joanna Johnson, is a massage therapist who lives in Creede, Colorado. After using her Gravity Pal® for only a few weeks Joanna shared with us a profound comment:

"The Gravity Pal® is surprisingly effective for something so seemingly benign."

Harnessing the law of gravity seems obvious. It's no surprise that inversion allows decompression.

So what caused Joanna to be surprised and, more importantly, why is the Gravity Pal® so surprisingly effective?

A Closer Look at the Difference Between Simple and Easy

We took an ancient idea of how to escape the effects of gravity. We then applied insights from Biomechanics, Physics and Physiology in an effort to create a way to go beyond back (or neck/shoulder/hip) pain and compression relief that also contributes to overall Wellness.

The closer we looked at the obvious angle issue we discovered many construction factors that either cause – or do not cause – new problems. And even after we had ironed out these construction factors we found many other new usage issues come into focus.

Even though the angle-height issue is obviously important because of the many impacts it has on the body, it became clear that looking at angle-height alone was like looking at building a car for speed without taking into account steering, brakes and what it's like to have – or not have – a windshield or a seat to sit on.

The most important of these several hidden issues – rarely discussed – is *method of use.* The more clearly we saw the bigger picture the more we keenly focused on the *method.* How should one use it?

Each of these issues: angle-height, construction factors and method of use, were going to impact the results we were looking for. We knew the table had to give an optimal experience for people to continue to use it as a Self-Care tool. The experience had to be *self-reinforcing,* otherwise people would not continue to use it.

Angle-Height First

First we looked at the effect we wanted and, importantly, the effects we did not want. We first focused on angle. We knew from experience we didn't want a higher one. But how low did we want to go, and how low was still going to be effective?

We knew we didn't want to strap in our feet, or trap them in some way, so how are we going to keep from sliding off? This required finding fabrics that are "slip resistant," which we discovered are not easy to find.

All of this brought into sharper focus the materials we were going to use as well as important physiological questions:

- ❖ *Is there a way to allow the spine to gently elongate and the upper body to be "more suspended" other than from the feet?*
- ❖ *What if we could devise a way so that the hips, while supported, could gently rotate and thus allow gravity to lengthen and decompress the spine?*
- ❖ *Would there be a way to create this so that the person felt relaxed, safe and secure?*

We knew we wanted to create a deeply restful experience the nervous system would *immediately* recognize as safe and secure. How to do that? This required a lot of testing, testing, and more testing.

Dozens of prototypes, well over 50, were built using various and sometimes wild designs.

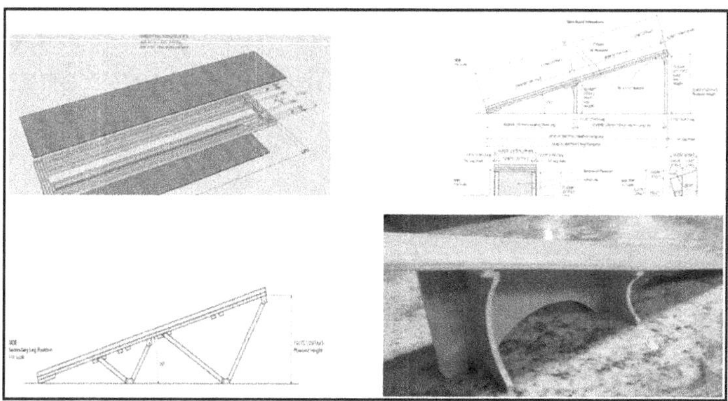

We tried different engineering concepts including cambering, span, SIPS (Structural Insulated Panels) and torsion boxes. We discovered that each material whether wood, metal, vinyl, or foam all come in multiple grades of strength, heaviness, lightness, breakability, slickness, stickiness, hardness, softness, flexibility, durability, availability and, of course, cost.

We tested many combinations of materials and angle-heights and even varied them by as little as 1/2" increments looking for that sweet spot where a foot strap was unnecessary.

When prototyping the foldable and portable Gravity Pal® *Traveler* we cut and recut the welds many times, sometimes as small as six-one-thousandths-of-an-inch, to get the pieces to fit together just-so.

Discovering the Common Problem
with Make-at-Home Inversion tables

In one of our earliest tests, we tried a very crude make-at-home option that we found in an older book about inversion.

It was suggested to simply staple some old carpet on a thick board and prop it up on a couch. We immediately learned:

1. **Bending.** A board of high quality 3/4" plywood, and even a thick 1 ½" board of solid oak, bent and sagged from the weight of our bodies.

   This bending phenomenon is a physics principle called "deflection." This became a focal point and key problem for us to solve.

   Lying on a sagging board created new pressure points particularly in our upper backs where the angle can cause a lot of additional pressure and pain.

   This had to be eliminated or neutralized or it would create more problems for people – the very opposite of what we wanted.

2. **Height.** Leaning the board up against a couch created an angle that was too high and uncomfortable.

3. **Slipping.** Even with the carpeting on the board, we were slipping off of it.

4. **Not Relaxing.** We felt more tense and in more pain – all of which were no good.

Based on our early experiences we developed the following "NO" checklist. We wanted:

❖ No or minimal board deflection/bending
❖ No creation of pressure points, and no new pains!
❖ No slipping off of it
❖ No immediate reaction of greater instability
   or tension either physically or psychologically

Instead we want

❖ A very solid feeling, immediately recognized by
   our nervous system, of being safe, secure and stable
❖ An experience so comfortable that the central
   nervous system can automatically let go and
   let all the tissues in the body relax

These last two points became the primary focus of our quest.

Muscle Guarding, a.k.a. the Startle Reflex

On one hand, harnessing the natural law of gravity seems obvious. It's no surprise that inversion allows for decompression.

However, when you invert the human physiology a number of things happen, some of which we have control over and some of which we do not, some physiological and some psychological.

Why psychological?

We have four ordinary vector relationships with gravity:

- ❖ Standing
- ❖ Walking
- ❖ Sitting
- ❖ Lying

Three of the four are more vertical and only one, lying down, is horizontal.

None are at an angle and none are lying backward on a slant with our head at a downward angle. None are inverted.

For some people the merest amount of slant, not to mention going upside down, can be emotionally uncomfortable. For some of these people, the disturbance can be mild, and for others it can be quite alarming.

For others a mild inversion can be immediately soothing and deeply relaxing. We've found this response is due to several factors, the angle being one of them.

But for all people their response is involuntary.

Inversion causes the human nervous system to react because our nervous system instantly knows that slanting or inversion is new, different, and out-of-the-ordinary.

This muscle guarding reaction is very easily triggered. It is automatic and part of our natural startle reflex. Faster than we can think about it we automatically recognize instability or "something new" and the nervous system – if it feels threatened – tightens up into a state of readiness and tension.

So our focus became:

A. How to take advantage of gravity in a positive way, and

B. How to *not* trigger this startle reflex or at least greatly minimize it

The Human Nervous System Knows It When it Experiences It

Our goal was to *not* turn the muscle guarding switch on. We sought to make the experience immediately restful – as recognized by the nervous system – and thus allow a quality compression release in the shortest possible time frame.

We looked at all the triggers of the startle reflex and we found that there are many things that can trigger this response both physiologically and psychologically:

<u>Physiological Triggers of Muscle Guarding</u>

- ❖ Pain of any kind
- ❖ Sudden strong sensations of heat, cold, noise or light
- ❖ Sudden imbalance like missing a stair-step

<u>Psychological Triggers of Muscle Guarding</u>

- ❖ Being tapped on one's shoulder unexpectedly
- ❖ Surprise or suddenness of any kind
- ❖ Hearing an unexpected word, phrase or news

Of course, we know that psychological reactions directly trigger physical reactions, like when someone yells *"BOO!"* behind your back.

Safe and Secure

When the body and mind sense everything is A.O.K. the nervous system relaxes and tells all the cells in the body that – for now – there is no threat or problem.

The most important observation we made is that when we feel safe and secure we do not experience sudden muscle guarding, and this sense of security coupled with short periods of inversion has potential cumulative benefits for us.

We knew that angle-height was one important factor. Finding a low enough angle where we would not trigger a muscle guarding reaction was critical.

We also knew we could not have any discomforts caused by bending boards or slipping surfaces.

Solving these problems, we believed, would allow tissues and fluids to be naturally released systemically.

The final result of our quest is what we now offer today as our line of Gravity Pal® low angle inversion tables and equally importantly, the method of using it.

Introduction to the *Gravity Pal Inversion Method*™

This method is based on three important observations:

1. **Shorter times are better.** Human beings are more likely to regularly do something if the amount of time required is the shortest possible.

2. **Natural Law.** The natural force of gravity has effects even at specific low angles.

3. **Regularity facilitates the opportunity of cumulative changes.**

A tool gets better results if it's used properly. We've found better results if a Gravity Pal® is used following our *Gravity Pal Inversion Method*™. This method has three main elements:

> 1. Short-duration
> 2. Low angle
> 3. Regular daily sessions

All three are important, but *regularity* is the most potent of all. It's obvious that regularly performing any positive action is part of any process of transformation.

A small-muscled person can remodel their body into that of a larger-muscled person by regularly exercising over time. Positive habits, regularly performed, matter *more* than each individual performance.

Although all the pieces and engineering of our tables create, in our opinion, a premium product of which we are very proud, the "secret sauce" behind Gravity Pal® low angle inversion tables is our method of using them: our combination of short, few-minute sessions, regularly experienced every day. In addition to these three main elements, there are other instructions we share only with our customers, that we believe greatly enhance and add efficacy to this unique method.

I would go so far as to say that our *Gravity Pal Inversion Method*™ may be the most important discovery we made while creating Gravity Pal®.

If you have another manufacturer's inversion table at home and can use it responsibly – meaning that using it will not create potential damage to your ankles, ligaments, or body in some way – then use it following this method of short durations, experienced regularly. I believe using <u>even just</u> these two elements of the *Gravity Pal Inversion Method*™ will greatly enhance your experience.

Of course, I continue to think that using this method along with a Gravity Pal® low angle inversion table provides the most superior experience. This is due to the many factors in our engineering that allow the user to experience a deep level of rest quickly, systemically and automatically. People who love their Gravity Pal tell us that lying on it produces an involuntary and natural response of deep rest. It is the repeated experience of this deep rest that we believe produces the results. We set up the correct conditions and nature (in this case, gravity) does the rest.

We consistently receive reports of a broad range of cumulative Wellness benefits that go beyond relief from back pain from those who have chosen to use a Gravity Pal® on a regular, daily basis of only a few minutes at a time. These include:

❖ Clearer thinking and better ability to focus
❖ More energy
❖ Less stress
❖ Faster recovery from intense exercise
❖ A New Form of Deep Systemic Rest — one person
   calls it his "meditation"

These effects are often reported after a few days or weeks of when they started their regular daily Gravity Pal® sessions.

Broad Range of Wellness Benefits Reported

As mentioned in the introduction of this book, I have an obvious bias and financial incentive for you to purchase a Gravity Pal® low angle inversion table. This is true and I hope you will visit our website (www.GravityPal.com) and consider purchasing one for yourself. On our site you'll find several testimonials from happy users. We continue to positive reports often. The two below are typical:

More Mental Clarity and Compression Relief

By Gary Greenfield, Florida

"I initially wanted a Gravity Pal® because I felt it would be a useful part of a holistic approach to alleviating chronic low-back pain. I wanted the benefit of gentle spinal decompression without any stress on the knees and ankles like typical inversion equipment. I have been using it twice-daily and look forward to the relief I get from each session. Another noticeable and unexpected side benefit is how it wakes my brain up. After three minutes on the Gravity Pal®, I definitely feel more alert and mentally smoother.

Two features I appreciate about the Gravity Pal® are its convenience and minimal footprint. Our small house is pretty crowded. I don't have room for even a small piece of equipment. But I can set up and put away my Gravity Pal® in literally ten seconds, and it fits neatly behind my office door. For all of these reasons, Gravity Pal® is very easy to fit into my busy and changeable schedule. A great product."

More Convenient and an Enjoyable Experience

By Anne Mitchell on Amazon.com

"This low angle inversion table does everything the full inversion tables do, without the necessity of strapping your ankles so that you will stay on it – or stretching your leg muscles so much that they may not return to their normal shape. I have used Gravity Boots, hanging upside down and full inversion tables which can cause physical discomfort and often require someone present so you can get off the table.

Most importantly, this product is well made and very, very comfortable; the pad is smooth and the inversion table seamless in spite of the folding edge. And without question, the customer service is the fastest, most complete and thoughtful anyone could ask for.

But why the low-angle table for me? It's more like yoga. The low angle gives me the tilt that puts my head down and legs up without strapping my ankles or stretching my muscles. Consistent use of the table in up to three minute intervals increases blood flow to the brain, shoulders and spinal cord....or so it seems to me. And increases my sense of wellbeing – I sense a rhythm to it. I'm high energy and this makes me quieter. And my feet, which carry the weight of my body are released from gravity – and love it.

The Gravity Pal® becomes my third piece of equipment, joining the Belicon rebounder and the Body Blade to provide a rounded physical exercise experience."

A New Form of Total Body Rest & Meditation

By Patrick Barron, Philadelphia, PA

This came about during a conversation I had with Pat after he had been using his Gravity Pal® about a year or so. Pat is 67 years old, quite fit and exercises regularly. He is retired from the US Air Force and once a year he hikes for a week in the Western US. When he's not actively golfing, fishing or doing something else he's chasing his grandchildren around.

Pat does not have chronic back issues. He is not debilitated by pain although his back sometimes gets stiff. He was attracted to Gravity Pal® because he heard of people reporting faster exercise recovery and clearer thinking from a few minutes of use.

I asked him in what ways he was finding it valuable. He told me, *"This is how I meditate."* I was quite surprised because I had not heard that from anyone before. He further explained, *"I feel a deep level of rest and after five minutes I'm ready to go. I try to do it every day and when I can't, I miss it."*

The above are typical of unsolicited comments we receive all the time. However, sometimes we hear of other benefits, such as a new ability to get back to sleep at night, better digestion or reduction of an unusual pressure or sensation in the abdomen.

Young & Old

We've been surprised by the young people who receive benefit from regular Gravity Pal® sessions. Our Amish upholsterer has a 12 year old daughter who told me she gets on it every night for 5 minutes because it helps her "back feel better."

We received an email from a mother in Austin, Texas who told us her high school-age daughter uses their Gravity Pal® to recover from her dance training and feels she could not keep up the rigorous pace of her schedule without it.

There are even college-aged "kids" we've heard from as well who, much to our surprise, experience chronic back pain their Gravity Pal® helps them manage.

One gentleman in his 50s told us he experienced relief from a chronic eyelid spasm that had bothered him his entire life. This went away after a couple of weeks of Gravity Pal® use and never came back.

Several persons have reported that their spinal alignment has improved and they need to see their chiropractor less often. So far we do not have research to verify that the spine is, in fact, becoming more aligned or straightened but would welcome a large-scale controlled study spanning several years so we can better understand these reported experiences.

In our opinion, these reports clearly indicate that something cumulative is producing these Wellness benefits. We believe this is due to people experiencing *short* periods of *low* angle inversion *regularly.*

Research is Needed

As of this writing, all we have to present as evidence are reports and testimonials. At this moment in history there exists no rigorous scientific research explaining why these effects occur.

We believe in good faith that these reported results are due to the regularity of people following a daily regimen simply because the reports are so consistent, but the scientist in us must readily admit that this is not proof.

In the Appendix of this book there is an *Invitation To Researchers* which presents a brief outline of our more technical ideas on why we believe low angle inversion and our *Gravity Pal Inversion Method™* deserves formal scientific research. We sincerely hope we receive inquiries from professional researchers to seriously study this important area.

Gravity Pal® is a Central Tool

In the previous chapter we pointed out that inversion is only one tool in our tool kit. Obviously, for me and for many others, regular daily sessions on a Gravity Pal® are a <u>central</u> tool that complements the other tools we may use.

More so, for me, it allows me to use other tools I could not use at all if I did not have my Gravity Pal®. I could not do all the other things I do without also having my Gravity Pal® readily available. But I am a serious case and for me all the Wellness benefits are secondary to the compression relief I repeatedly need to have.

But for many other people the compression relief is secondary, or tertiary, or not that important at all.

Many people tell us they are primarily motivated to use their Gravity Pal® for a variety of other Wellness reasons that are important to them. They want a quick way to rest, or to increase their energy, a way to sharpen their mental clarity, experience better digestion, improved beauty or several other things that are important to them.

These people have inspired me. Those who are motivated beyond relief from back pain because they experience a broader spectrum of Wellness benefits – and have seen the results they seek from using their Gravity Pal® – are the reason I continue to believe Gravity Pal® will become a widely used tool.

People will use it because it works for them.

Tools are like that. Some you need more often than others and will rely on more. Some tools are more central to our health and Wellness.

CHAPTER 9

HOW I BUILT MY TOOLKIT & HOW YOU CAN BUILD ONE THAT WORKS

The Key Importance of Regaining Balance

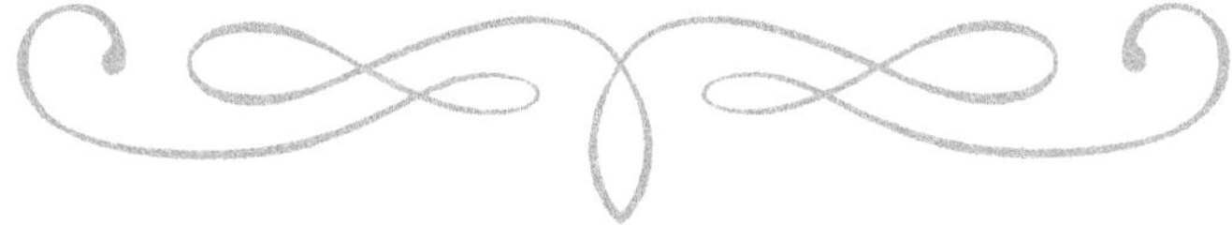

You may recall from Chapter 5 that, according to Ayurveda, the root cause of diseases are impurities and imbalances.

I left you hanging in Chapter 5 when I said there are several strategies for regaining balance that we'd cover in Chapter 9 – and here we are.

The focal point of Chapters 5 and 6 were to emphasize that regaining balance is of primary importance to our health and Self-Care process.

As you read through this chapter you'll be introduced to several different ideas, strategies, modalities, and tools that I use. <u>Every one of them</u>, every tool in my toolkit I chose to help me regain balance in various ways.

Please keep that in mind when you're building your own toolkit. All the various pieces can be selected with this one question in mind: *can this help me gain and regain balance in a way that I need it?*

Balance – as we've been talking about it – may seem elusive, even impossible. There are so many moving parts! How can we be in balance? And even more so, how can we regain balance?

Let me make this clear. The better term is plural: balance*s*.

There's a myriad of ways we become imbalanced: we get tired, hungry, and dirty. Emotionally, we sometimes feel several varieties of imbalance: anger, fear, doubt, uncertainty. Sometimes our minds are clear but other times we're foggy. Our bodies can feel just fine or we have aches and pains – some severe or chronic – where we certainly don't feel balanced.

Regaining Balance is a Constant Process

Actually, regaining balance is a constant *series* of processes.

There's an old saying, *"Living in a human body is like living in a house on fire."*

No kidding!

Life is like this. You'll recall that *Provocation* is the second of the Six Stages of Disease we covered in Chapter 5. I referred to provocation as *life and living.*

Life and living is a constant process of dealing with – and choosing to either correct or ignore – impurities and imbalances we accumulate every single day.

Skip a meal? We get hungrier. Skip a night's sleep? We are very tired. Gaining balance and regaining balance is our job – our #1 job as humans.

But when it comes to pain – acute or chronic, we need to pay special attention. What, in addition to a healthy lifestyle will help *me* – especially when I'm in pain?

Following the four *Dance Steps to Wellness* in Chapter 6 will be a big help. This chapter on building your toolkit will help. Everything I've shared can help.

The "Due North" on our Wellness Compass is **balance and regaining it**.

Keep yourself focused on balance and regaining it and you'll make progress in your life.

Let's Get Started

When I first imagined this book I wanted it to be valuable to everyone who wants to escape back pain and create greater Wellness in their life. I know for certain that I've achieved this for myself to some measure. However, I can't guarantee it to you or any other person. All I can tell you is my story and hope that it both inspires you and assists you to work to achieve this for yourself to whatever degree you can.

I've achieved great progress which lasted for months, and experienced setbacks that, at times, were very discouraging and lasted for months as well.

So, Look at the Trend

Life goes on. Sometimes it is more rewarding and sometimes it is more challenging than other times. Sometimes it's all about celebrating.

In 2012, in celebration of my 61st birthday, I was leading an 80 foot rock climb in a canyon about 30 miles north of Ojai, California with my mentor and friend Matthew Fienup. It was a moderately difficult (5.7) crack climb and I completed it without too much trouble.

After finishing the climb and rappelling down we chatted with two younger guys I would guess to be in their early 30s who were waiting to climb after us.

One of these fellows mentioned a more difficult climb they'd done a week before in Joshua Tree National Park, which is about 200 miles east of where we were climbing that day.

I recognized that route from a previous trip with Matthew and asked them,

"Did you climb in the trough or climb out on the rail?"

Surprised I knew that climbing route they said, *"The trough."*

Matthew piped up, *"Michael climbed it out on the rail and he's over 60 years old."*

I admit that I enjoyed Matthew bragging about me since the "rail" was considered a more challenging climb. One of the waiting climbers spoke up,

"Gee," he said, *"I've got to tell my dad to get off the couch."* (ha!)

I tell you that story because it was a high point of celebration for me. I was flying high in 2012.

But in September 2014 I was back on my knees and it was many months before I could even *think* about rock climbing again.

Always Look at the Trend – the Longer the Better

When I look back at where I was in 2001, 2005, 2012, 2014, and today I can plot a definite upward trend – with a lot of setbacks along the way.

Here's the point: the four steps of Wellness are a *dance.* Sometimes you're coping, sometimes you're overcoming obstacles, and sometimes you're celebrating. Most of the time you're at Step #2: *working on making progress.* This chapter is mostly about this second step.

You'll achieve your upward trend by keeping focused on improving and making progress, and by believing that you can do it even when you're in the stages of coping and overcoming obstacles.

The *3rd Dance Step of Wellness* of overcoming obstacles, I believe, is where the hardest work is done. When you experience a setback it is both emotionally and physically like sliding down the mountain you worked very hard to climb. Overcoming obstacles, as I have come to know, may very well happen again and again, and if that's the case you've got to get comfortable with it. Getting through the stages of coping and overcoming obstacles is really the foundation of your Wellness plan.

So before we get to the rest of the toolkit let's cover three related areas intrinsic to both coping and overcoming obstacles. Understanding how these fit together will help you and your team create a pain management strategy:

* Knowing when to call for help
* Understanding your experience and its potential causes
* Defining pain and how to communicate with your doctor about it

Know When to Call for Help

The first rule of being a healthcare provider is to *do no harm.* This is even more important for Self-Care. There is a point when you must call for help. Also, the first team member you need to create is the doctor or therapist who will be your go-to person when an urgent need arises.

When serious pain manifests don't wait. We know that complications and even chronic pain can soon follow. Here you have to help your doctor/therapist help you. Sounds easy, but it's more complicated than you may realize.

The Problems

Pain can have many causes and it can have a great number of ways in which it is described. When you show up at your doctor's office and say, *"I'm in pain"* the doctor has to try to divine a great number of things. The most important question, of course, is what is causing the pain. Simply asking that question opens up a number of potential avenues of inquiry.

Understanding Your Experience

You want to become a responsible General Contractor for your pain management strategy. What follows is a different kind of descriptive process that you may find both useful when talking to your doctor or therapist. The more you can tell them, the more they can help you.

What is Causing the Pain?

Broadly speaking we can say that most pains are caused or influenced by four factors:

1. Compression

2. Inflammation and degeneration

3. Energy depletion

4. Systemic issues

Compression

How much is compression a factor in your pain? We could make a broad statement that, in various ways, the effects of gravity may be a factor in many kinds of chronic pain – especially back pain.

Compression issues may arise from repetitive motions, postures, or internal pressures on localized tissues where the muscle fibers have become shortened. If you have internal scarring, like in the case of endometriosis, the gravitational effects of day-to-day living may be contributing to your daily discomfort.

For you, the impact of compression may be a lesser factor, or it may be a primary factor. In either case, it is worthwhile to evaluate if obtaining regular relief from gravity and compression may be of assistance to your situation.

Inflammation and Degeneration

We could say that there is good inflammation and bad inflammation. Fevers can protect us or can kill us; the right "dosage" of inflammation is important.

Really bad inflammation is the kind that wears out tissue-fibers prematurely. Think of it as friction – like a slow burn – that degenerates the tissues over time.

When I was a young man I had a brief stint selling *Fuller Brush Products*[19] door-to-door. The pitch for their best-selling laundry soap involved a demonstration with two clear plastic jars of soapy water. One of the jars was filled with our colorless "low suds"

---

[19] Established in 1906, Fuller Brush Products is an American Institution. I was proud to sell their products. www.fullerproducts.com

product which we compared to a blue-colored, nationally-advertised TV brand with "high suds." The TV brand also had a lot of flakes that swirled around like you'd see in a snow globe whenever I'd shake it up.

I would ask the prospective buyer, *"Do you wonder how those little holes appear in your family's t-shirts, causing them to wear out prematurely?"*

They would always say, *"Yes."*

While shaking the two jars side by side I would tell them,

"This national brand contains an additive that causes the soap to foam and suds but really doesn't help clean the clothes. Worse, this additive is not fully rinsed out and leaves a residue that causes clothes to wear out prematurely.

"Our product doesn't have that additive."

Because our soap did not have these additives and actually got the clothes cleaner (and was much less expensive) it was one of our most popular products. People would quickly see the value in not having their fabrics wear out so fast.

What Reduces the Wear and Tear on Our Human Fabrics?

Of course, our human "fabrics" (fascia, muscle, ligaments, tendons, skin, bone and every other kind of tissue in the body) are far more complex than what our t-shirts are made of. Plus, our human fabrics actually regenerate via the process of remodeling. Our fabrics are constantly being replaced by new fabric cells. However, chronic inflammation is like having a "high suds" additive stuck in our body and, over time, this chronic inflammation can prematurely wear out – degenerate – our tissues and cause conditions such as arthritis and other painful ailments throughout the body.

This requires that we quiet down the inflammation causes and responses in the body that are creating excessive fire alarms throughout it. This may be aided by diet and supplements.[20]

Energy Depletion and Tissues Feeling Weaker

Muscle soreness after exercise is a simple example of energy depletion. It is often corrected by proper hydration, good nutrition, and rest.

However, repetitive energy depletion without adequate recovery can increase tissue weaknesses, cause inflammation, and become the root of bigger problems. This can come from sitting too long, standing too long, or taxing the body in repetitive patterns over and over.

Office Work or Physical Labor Can Cause It

One would think that people would simply back off, take breaks and give their bodies time to repair. However, it is common for us to see the effects of simply not alternating rest and activity in the right balance.

Some physically demanding professions can cause longer-term energy depletion and directly cause compression issues, greater inflammation, and degeneration in the tissues – all at the same time.

---

[20] Products that I use can be found in the *Resource Guide.*

The best kept (dirty) secret in the massage profession is that many massage therapists do not receive regular massages themselves. As a result, there are some massage therapists who are working while injuring themselves, which is both ironic and tragic.

Fortunately, many massage therapists have discovered using Gravity Pal® low angle inversion tables for 1-2 minutes between their client sessions. This allows their system a quick opportunity to rest, repair and restore energy in the system. I look forward to the day when Gravity Pals are in most warehouses, docks, building sites, and other workplaces where people can receive a meaningful amount of rest and recovery in only 1-2 minutes – whenever they want.

Systemic Pain

One example of this is *Fibromyalgia* which can present a broad range of symptoms including pain, fatigue, and sleeplessness that often befuddle physicians to identify the root cause. We do know the fascia and muscle fibers of people with this syndrome are chronically shortened, which is considered one cause of the widespread pain.

Other, more serious conditions, like Multiple Sclerosis and Parkinson's Disease can also create widespread systemic pain.

However, on a more minor level, we could simply have a nutritional imbalance or feel achy "all over" due to excessive fatigue. Whether the causes are very serious or minor, there are many ways to benefit the individual and help to reduce systemic symptoms. These include various herbal supplements, warm salt baths, inversion and gentle non-force therapies like massage, Craniosacral Therapy, and Zero Balancing. The broader the systemic issue, the broader the approach may need to be.

Defining Pain and How to Communicate with your Doctor

The Problem: Everyone's Pain is Different

Doctors have faced this quandary forever – how to "feel" their patients pain. Words can only go so far. They know they cannot truly feel it, because pain is always a subjective experience.

Nevertheless, medical science has made many serious attempts to find a way for patients to effectively communicate with the doctors about pain. Since 1975, the McGill Pain Questionnaire (MPQ) remains one of the most widely-used methods of describing and measuring pain using subjective descriptors of quality and intensity. Even though it was considered a breakthrough, the essential problem remains obvious: the questionnaire tries to translate what is nearly impossible to.

Because of this, conversations between patients and doctors can be very frustrating for them both.

You already know that pain is a subjective experience and that it comes in many experiential flavors. It can be anywhere from mild to unbearable. Like you, I've experienced all kinds of pain – like biting, prickly, burning, stinging, aching, throbbing, shooting, intense, radiating, and exhausting.

I offer you a few words which you and your doctor may find useful. They cover five areas: priority, functionality, intensity, location, and descriptors. Your doctor is used to hearing about the last three but I have found it valuable to communicate the first two, priority and functionality, to my doctors to help them better understand the experience I'm having.

Priority
Dangerous, Potentially Dangerous, and Not Dangerous

Functionality
Greatly Disruptive, Disruptive and Mildly Disruptive to your activity

Intensity
Severe, Intermittently Severe, Bad, and Somewhat Tolerable

Location
Generally worse (Here), Travels from (Here to Here), Radiates from (Here to Here), and Right Here

Descriptors
Use as many adjectives to describe it as needed.

Write these down and take them to your doctor who may find this additional information useful. Keep a copy for yourself when assessing your future progress.

Building your Toolkit – A Story on Getting Organized

There's an old story about an adult daughter visiting her professor father who was a researcher known for working on many projects. One day, the professor had to be away and the daughter thought she would help her dad by organizing his very messy office. She spent the whole day sorting and filing the many stacks of books and file folders that were willy-nilly all over the place. She was quite proud of how clean and tidy it all was when she finished.

When the professor returned he was aghast – and quite angry – that he couldn't find anything! You see, he had everything organized according to *priority* and his daughter had just assumed that the best way to file everything was *alphabetically.*

The problem with organizing is that each of us conceives of it one way, but others may actually conceive of – and do it – another way. Please don't let this be a problem for you. Don't over-think or try to organize building your toolkit just because it is my way. **Your way is what works for you.**

It's wonderful to be organized but more important to *act.*

Stay Focused on the *Doing – Today*

Ask yourself every day, "What am I going to do *today?"* Then make sure you get that done before you go to bed that night. Make it a daily commitment to do <u>something</u> every day and mix it up; weights, walking, yoga, Gravity Pal®, etc.

Every, every, every day do *something* – at least one thing.

The progress you'll make is built on taking action, on what you *do.* Of all the messages and lessons I have learned about Self-Care, this is the most important of all.

I'm going to share tools that I use today and some I've used in the past that were critical for coping and for making progress. I'll share items that you too can use for your toolkit.

Of course, I'm not providing medical advice and I'm not saying that you'll obtain the results I or others I may refer to have achieved. In fact, there are things I'm going to recommend, but because of your particular situation, some of you absolutely should not do.

But there are two things you absolutely must do:

1. You have to pick something to do every day that will help you cope or help you make progress. It may only take 1 to 3 minutes, but every day commit to getting that done.

2. You must enlist at least one doctor or licensed healthcare provider to be on your Self-Care team. This is the first thing that goes into your toolkit.

First Thing in Your Toolkit – Your Self-Care Team

In my case, I have four on my Self-Care team besides me – my primary care M.D. who is also my 5-Element Acupuncturist, a chiropractor who is also trained as a Registered Nurse, a licensed massage therapist who is also certified in Zero Balancing and Myofascial Therapy, and a certified fitness trainer. It helps if they all know and respect one another; if you can arrange that, all the better.

As to the rest of the tools, modalities, and strategies that I will share with you, I want you to apply common sense and openly discuss everything you are doing with all of your team members, keeping all of them informed of each new idea you have, reaction to it, and new modality you are considering starting – and each modality you have chosen to stop. Openly discuss what is going on for you. Each one wants to assist you the best way they can. They all will have something to share and their perspectives are important.

If you enlist a health professional that does not seem that interested in all this kind of detail, then fire them and find another to replace them – that is what a General Contractor needs to do.

I see each of my professionals on a pretty regular schedule. My trainer and massage therapist I see every week or two. My chiropractor I see about every month or so. My MD/Acupuncturist I see every couple of months or so. I provide a report about my experiences with each other team member every time I see any one of them.

The Key Reason This Kind of Sharing is Important

Whenever I've encountered an obstacle or a setback, having each member of my team know what is going on for me allows them – through me – to make suggestions about the other modalities. This is valuable to each and every one of them, and to me in particular.

For example, I've told my chiropractor and massage therapist that I overdid it with my weight training by overdoing my Sumo Squats at home, which created unwanted symptoms in my hips and lower back. This kind of information was very valuable to both my massage therapist and chiropractor who, armed with this detail, were able to assist me to return to full functionality much faster as a result.

In another case I told my fitness trainer how my massage therapist and chiropractor – in combination – had helped me free up my shoulder. As a result, my fitness trainer was able to devise a remedial program that helped my shoulder improve very quickly.

It has also happened that I saw my M.D. regarding a medical problem and he had a suggestion for one of my other team members. It was my M.D. who introduced me to my chiropractor in the first place. Their professional relationship, working together, is how my team really got started.

You can see from these examples that in building your toolkit, building your team is a central part of the process.

Second Thing in Your Tool Kit – Modalities

A modality is a method of therapeutic approach and there are a lot of them. We are going to look at two types: Self-Care and Professional Care.

Modalities include things that you can do alone, all by yourself, or they may be something that requires a professional, like chiropractic, massage or Zero Balancing.

Some things like Pilates, weight training, meditation, and yoga you may be able to do by yourself – alone – after you've received some training.

Determining which modalities are best for you is a dynamic process where you're always evaluating, evaluating, evaluating the effectiveness of your modalities and service providers.

Here are the modalities I regularly use and notice it when I miss any of them for one reason or another. More information on each can be found in the *Resource Guide.*

- ❖ Four Minute Miracle
- ❖ Low angle inversion
- ❖ Weight training
- ❖ Transcendental Meditation Technique
- ❖ 5-Element Acupuncture
- ❖ Chiropractic
- ❖ Dead Sea Salt Baths
- ❖ Massage & Zero Balancing

Other Modalities

For some people, simply walking will be a modality in their toolkit. When I was in my coping stage, walking was an important method of therapy for me – now it's a joyful activity. Before my spinal fusion surgery walking was nearly impossible and was a very big goal when I couldn't even walk short distances without lying down, sobbing with pain.

Now I do a great many things I could not do before; I walk a lot, I rock climb on my barn and sometimes out on real rock, I help with the gardening, I carry stuff up and down stairs. All of these, at one time, were out of the question. That is why I think that everything you do can become a part of your "modalities."

When you start this process there are things that may be more challenging than perhaps later. My hope for you is that you will be able to do each of them more regularly and with greater ease.

Make Sure Everything You Do Is:

❖ **Attractive** Each modality should be attractive to you and, if at all possible, fun in some way. Having a great Pilates or fitness trainer can really help. At very least, it should not be repellant to you or arduous for you to do.

❖ **Convenient** *How much time is all this is going to take?* My answer: as little as possible! If you pick the right modalities, they should only take a few minutes that you can easily find. Adding these few minutes into your daily and weekly routines should leverage your time and make your activity so much more rewarding that you'll have more time to enjoy and celebrate life. After all, that is why we do this.

❖ **<u>Sustainable</u>** You should do what you can regularly sustain. Keep in focus what is effective that you can perform regularly. The key to progress — and cumulative results — is sustainable regularity. If you like it, it's convenient, and actually leverages your time, you are more likely to be able to sustain and derive the cumulative benefits potentially possible.

❖ **<u>No Rough Stuff</u>** I believe, whenever possible, to only use non-force modalities rather than "rough stuff" type therapies. I've been to far too many therapists who want me to be extra macho, grit my teeth and let them bore into my body in a very intrusive and painful way. There is a time and place to endure short moments of discomfort in some legitimate therapeutic processes, but most of the time it's just not necessary, and is even counterproductive.

All the modalities I use are non-force or minimal-force approaches that focus on harnessing the laws of nature to my advantage. Even the deep-tissue massage work that I receive every week is done in a non-force way. If you find a massage therapist who says deep tissue work cannot be performed without pain and discomfort, find yourself another massage therapist because I assure you it can be done.

⊙ You should work within your comfort range and only test the outside edges of your tolerance levels

⊙ The only kind of pain that may be okay is the soreness that comes from exercise, but again, always within your ability to tolerate it. You have to be the judge.

❖ **No Feather-Shaking Modalities Welcome** The term "non-force" for some people conjures up ideas of voodoo and other patently non-scientific approaches. We want real results. We want meaningful effects in people's lives using modalities that deliver results through the cumulative exposure to these modalities.

❖ **Start Off Slow** Be realistic about your fitness level and try not to overdo it, especially at the beginning. Slow and steady wins the race. When you overdo it, back off and start over, slowly.

❖ **Let Your Plan Evolve as You Do** Pay attention to what works and what you like. Keep it fresh. Change the order of things. Even if it's working for you, don't get bored. Stay flexible and open to new things. This is much easier if you work with your team to help you keep it evolving.

Many of you already have a number of modalities in motion. If you're starting from scratch, just pick two modalities for your toolkit at first. Pick one thing you can do every day and one more thing you'll do at least once a week. Once you start a rhythm of sustainable *doing,* the momentum of greater Wellness and living better will carry you forward.

Third Thing in Your Tool Kit – Free Stuff, Equipment & Supplies

My support tools fall into one of three categories:

❖ Free Stuff
❖ Low Tech Stuff (that is relatively free-per-use)
❖ Investments that tend to be expensive, but are worth it

I select tools from these categories based on whether they have immediate relief potential or cumulative relief potential – or, if possible, both. I want every tool to be something valuable that most likely I will use and will be very convenient for me.

When it comes to equipment, I also want as few items as possible. I have seen far too many people who purchase unnecessary tools which makes them somehow think they're doing something for themselves when they're only cluttering up their life.

I recommend the criteria *Most Likely to Use* should be your primary selection criterion that overrides all others.

Free Stuff

I have seven things on my *Free Stuff* list.

The first four are *Walking, Ice, Cool-to-Cold Showers* and *"Legs Up on the Couch While Lying on the Floor,"* which is an alternative if you do not have an inversion table available to you.

The fifth is a creative option of using a hill or outdoor incline. One of my friends told me he does this when he is out on long walks and needs an *"inversion break."* Although it may not be available to the average person, it demonstrates how creative you can become once you're aware of the cumulative benefits of regularly experiencing low angle inversion.

The last two items on the *Free Stuff* list require more information. Therefore I'll give you a brief introduction to them below. In the Appendix I've prepared more detailed information about each of them which I hope you'll read later.

One is a powerful discovery I've made called the *4 Minute Miracle.* Finally, I'll briefly introduce *Drinking Water as a Key to Pain Management & Wellness.*

All seven of these *Free Stuff* items are simple and powerful options for your toolkit.

<u>Walking</u>

Here is a fun story. I was attending a conference where we sat for hours on uncomfortable chairs. One fellow attendee who knew I was a massage therapist asked if I would take a look at his newly-aching back. He said it was really bothering him, so much so that he thought he might not be able to continue with the conference.

I said to him, *"Let's take a walk and talk about it."* After about ten minutes of walking I asked him how his back was feeling. To his amazement he said it felt completely better!

Sometimes, simply walking is all we need to do to alleviate minor – or even stronger – back pain. It's free and worth trying out. Remember, everyone's pain is subjective. My conference friend was quite disturbed by his painful back. For him, and for many others, a short walk can bring the relief needed.

Walking, all by itself, can be a great tool that everyone should embrace. We should take a lesson from John Adams, the second President of the United States. He walked three miles every single day, and he also lived for 86 years when the average person never lived past 50. I'm convinced that regular walks can also assist your overall health – specifically the health of your back, hips and joints. Try it out. Put it on your list to walk for 10 minutes a day if you can spare it. If not, always take the *longer way around* throughout your day.

Ice

Inflammation, depending on where it is, responds well to ice. Often used for joint injuries to reduce swelling, it can also be useful to reduce higher orders of pain you may experience.

If you have sharp, needle-like back pains, as I have had from time to time, taking a bag of frozen peas from the freezer may be just the ticket to quiet them down. It always works for me and it breaks the pain cycle, which sometimes is all I need to achieve immediate relief.

A zip-lock bag of ice can also be used. Most people require a cloth between the bag and their skin for comfort. In that case, use the thinnest cloth you have. Personally, I've developed a tolerance for the frozen peas to be placed directly on my skin with no cloth between. That is, even for me, a big eye-opening experience! But it's amazing how quickly I can adjust to it.

Please Note: I am not recommending you attempt such a "Viking Experience" as to not use a cloth between your skin and the ice bag, but if you do be ready – it is bracing! In either event, you should keep the ice on the area for a maximum of 10 minutes at a time. If you want, you can remove it for 10 minutes and then put it back on for 10 more minutes.

Cool-to-Cold Showers (and how to take them)

Many health enthusiasts endorse cold showers and many claim it reduces chronic pain and makes the body healthier in a number of ways. My research indicates that this is still a controversial subject. I think one reason for the controversy is that it only focuses on *COLD* showers or baths.

Those with high blood pressure are warned to avoid shocking themselves with cold water, and for good reason! Dr. Andrew Weil says, *"I advise against it for anyone who has high blood pressure.*

Low temperatures (including cold weather) constrict blood vessels. As a result, blood pressure rises because more pressure is needed to force blood through narrowed blood vessels." [21]

On the other side of the argument, you'll find many websites and articles that list a large number of benefits from regularly taking cold showers, asserting that they:

1. Decrease chronic pain

2. Increase fat loss

3. Improve lymphatic circulation, thereby enhancing immunity against infections

4. Improve hormonal activity and glandular health (thyroid, adrenals, ovaries/testes)

5. Improve mood and can reduce symptoms of depression

6. Normalize blood pressure and improve blood circulation

7. Detoxify the body

8. Reduce insomnia

9. Rejuvenate and tone the skin

10. Improve temperature regulation, reducing excessive sweating and chronically cold hands and feet, and more [22]

---

[21] https://www.drweil.com/health-wellness/body-mind-spirit/hair-skin-nails/
are-cold-showers-good-for-you

[22] http://www.cold-showers.com/a-doctors-view-on-cold-showers

So, who's right?

First, I'm only going to tell you what I do and what I have found in my personal experience. It is up to you to decide whether or not to try them out.

I like taking *cool-to-cold* showers every day, and I think they've reduced chronic pain levels in my body. I also believe they help me with fat burning, which is always welcome. So as far as I'm concerned, it's worth doing.

Second, I'm not going to endorse just-cold-only showers for everyone. There are those of you who may love them – have at it! But they are not for me.

Back in the 1970s, I spent one winter in Switzerland going to school and living in a building that had no hot water. I had to take cold baths – *really* cold baths – for several months. I used to draw out the water the night before so it wouldn't be so brutally cold by morning. When I awoke I would muster the courage to face that tub again. I'd step in, bar of soap in hand, sit down (always a shock) splash water all over me, stand up – shaking and shivering – soap up all over, then plunge into the cold water for a very quick rinse and get the heck out of that tub.

I can tell you that I never liked the experience. But then a funny thing happened. When I came back to the USA I discovered I really didn't like hot, or even warm showers anymore. Over time I found that cool-to-cold works just great for me and I really like them. But too cold, *"No Thank You!"*

There are many people who think the whole idea of cold showers is nuts. And, objectively, I totally see their point. I am against shocking the nervous system and have experienced the middle ground that I'll present below.

I hope you'll discover for yourself whether cool-to-cold, or even just cold showers help you or not.

How to Take Cool-to-Cold Showers

Start with your normal shower temperature and slowly turn it down until it STARTS to feel a little cool to you. Then proceed with your shower as normal.

Soon you'll notice that you've gotten used to the less-hot temperature. Now turn the temperature down just a little further. You'll soon find you've gotten used to that temperature and can again make it even a little cooler.

End your shower with what I call the "Goose Bump" temperature – which is another level cooler until you *start* to feel goose bumps.

Finish rinsing and you're done.

Next time you shower, try starting with a little cooler temperature and proceed to make it a little cooler again and again. Soon you'll find that you are starting with a cool shower and ending with an even cooler shower on a regular basis.

When I step out of the shower I feel very refreshed but am not shivering. My skin feels cool to the touch but I quickly warm up. In the winter I dress warmly anyway. But I also like to sit in an infrared sauna for 15 to 20 minutes as well to "warm up my bones" every few days. Over time you'll find that alternating intentionally warming and cooling your body may be something you like which adds to your sense of Wellness.

One more tip: if you take the warm salt bath suggestion that I will be presenting later in this chapter, end it with a slightly cooler – but still-warm rinse. What you'll find is that you can get goose bumps even when you're rinsing in warm-ish water. This is because your body is reacting to the contrasting temperature your body which is creating the goose bumps.

If you try out cool-to-cold showers you may notice that you not only tolerate colder water temperatures, but you can actually grow to like them. Follow your own experience. Like all the tools you will gather, take it step by step and you'll find out what works for you.

Legs Up On the Couch

I add this because it is a way to almost create an inversion effect for the body. Even though the back is flat on the floor and the lower legs are flat on the couch cushions, the back is allowed to relax and the elevated legs stimulate a large amount of lymph to flow upward in the body, towards the heart.

This is a far cry from the effects one would have on a Gravity Pal® low angle inversion table, but it's free and it does provide some relief. In any case, it is a valuable tool to keep and to use.

If you choose to do this here are three tips:

1. Scoot your butt as close to the couch as you can, and

2. Once your legs are up on the couch, only lay there for 1-2 minutes, especially if you haven't done this before or are not doing it regularly, and

3. Roll off and lay on the floor for at least 30 seconds after you're finished

Finally, please keep this option in mind when you do the *4 Minute Miracle* which we'll talk about soon.

Find a Hill & Lay Down On It – Getting Creative
My friend Paul is a retired, 69-year-old graphic artist who's a serious woodworking hobbyist. Paul volunteers with the Boy Scouts helping kids working on their woodworking merit badges. He's one of my favorite people and uses his Gravity Pal® regularly.

One day we were chatting about how it naturally happens to Gravity Pal® users, when they find it unavailable for some reason, that they miss it and wish there was some way they could get in a few minutes of low angle inversion.

Paul then told me his unique creative solution.

Every Saturday he walks the beautiful 16-mile nature trail that loops around our little rural town of Fairfield, Iowa.

Paul tells me he's found two places along the trail where there's a slight incline. When he arrives to these spots he lays down on the ground – head pointing downhill – and takes a few minute, low angle inversion break.

Paul said these little breaks make walking the trail more comfortable – and possible – for him.

This story goes to show that once you get into the rhythm of regular low angle inversion sessions you'll look for ways to make them happen for you when you're away from your Gravity Pal®.

This was a big reason behind the development of our foldable and portable Gravity Pal® *Traveler* low angle inversion table.

We've had many people purchase two Gravity Pals® and ship one to a relative or friend's house they might be visiting for a while. It's also why we developed the Gravity Pal® Airline Checkable Luggage Case so people could just take theirs wherever they may go. Our portable Gravity Pal® *Travelers* have indeed traveled the world over – from Bali, to Europe and beyond.

Candidly, the primary reason we developed the Gravity Pal® *Traveler* was for me. I find it difficult to travel without one. My personal Self-Care program greatly benefits from using my Gravity Pal® a minimum of twice a day – especially when I'm traveling. I'm a lot more comfortable – and can quickly and easily regain a state of greater comfort, because I keep mine handy. When I travel, the first thing I do when I arrive is set up my *Traveler* and lay on it for 1 to 3 minutes.

Sure, it's great to get all those cumulative benefits from regular sessions I talk about throughout this book, but sometimes all we want – and need – is relief.

And just like Paul walking on his trail, sometimes all I need is the relief I get in those few minutes.

4 Minute Miracle

In the *Appendix* I present this brief, super-easy-to-do program I developed and do every single day.

It's a light exercise series that takes four minutes that virtually anyone in any health condition can do. Regularly doing it has numerous potential benefits, not only for back pain or other compression-related relief, but overall Wellness. Check it out. I recommend it as one of the first things you – and everyone – put in their toolkit.

<u>Drinking Water as a Key to Pain Management & Wellness</u>

Of all the things you can add to your toolkit, drinking and *absorbing* (a key word) the proper amount of water – every day – is the most essential of the Free Stuff.

This is a big and surprisingly controversial topic. I've devoted several pages in the Appendix on how drinking and absorbing the proper amount of water every day impacts pain management and long-term Wellness.

Even if you're already drinking all the water you think you need, I guarantee you'll learn new tips and gain a better understanding why drinking and *absorbing* water is an essential part of everyone's toolkit. Please check it out.

Low-Tech Stuff

I have only four low-tech tools that I regularly use and widely recommend: *Weights, Warm Dead Sea Salt Baths,* a *Q-Flex* and, of course a *Gravity Pal*® low angle inversion table.

There are many other items that could be added to this list of low-tech stuff that I see other people using. For example, my wife regularly uses a half-roll of hard foam. She says that 1 minute on that really helps her back and hips. Personally, I cannot tolerate it and am happy it works for her.

I have friends who use yoga blocks and straps for stretching. One friend gave me a present of a ball in a sock (I think it's a hard rubber squash ball) he claims gives him immediate relief whenever a certain part of his back bothers him. Another friend duct-taped two tennis balls together and uses that to help him with his chronic back pain, which he also gave me as a gift. I have used all of these and they all have value, but they are not my go-to items. You, too, will find yours. Stay open and experiment.

Some of my clients swear by mini-trampolines. Many of these are relatively inexpensive, however, some can be found as $20 versions and others as $300 versions.

The purpose of this section is not to provide a review on any of these items, but to point out that inexpensive, low-tech tools are out there. Some you can make yourself. Many of these can assist you in your efforts to immediately reduce pain and improve systemic balance and Wellness.

Rather than comment on all of these options I recommend you follow these principles:

1. Pick Modalities – methods of therapy – first

2. Add as few pieces of equipment as you can. Keep it simple.

3. Think longer-term

4. Network with your team and other Self-Care-focused people to see what they are using. Ask to borrow their stuff, try it out and see what works for you.

A Word About Spending Money

Many things are free or nearly free. Brad Johnson's book *"Extraordinary Strength"* outlines a process that uses old pieces of PVC pipe, scrap 2'x4' boards, and old golf balls as tools. There are creative ways you may find to not spend money. If you can do that, by all means do so.

However, as we know, virtually everything costs money and we shouldn't let money be a barrier from selecting valuable tools for ourselves. If your budget is tight, it's valuable to go through a three-step process.

First, just look at what a tool can potentially do for you. Second, figure out what it may cost you if you were to use it every day over time. You want to know its *Cost-Per-Use.*

Even though something may cost you hundreds of dollars upfront, it may only cost you 10¢ a day to use over time – and wind up saving you many thousands of dollars in the long run.

It's important to ask yourself what less-painful days and nights are worth to you. This is not a dollar figure, per se, but in the end is a KEY aspect of the decision. The right tool can create a great deal of comfort and Wellness leverage for you, which in turn may make you more productive in life.

The right tools can help you not only maintain balance and make progress more quickly but also to overcome obstacles and regain a healthier state of balance more quickly. Look at each tool, each piece of equipment and ask yourself if it has the potential to play an essential role to your long-term Wellness process.

This is also a very valuable exercise when you evaluate the cost-per-use for various modalities where you perform some of it on your own and some with a trainer. This also would apply when a larger upfront investment is required, like learning the Transcendental Meditation Technique, which, once learned, you can derive significant benefit from every single day – for the rest of your life.[23]

---

[23] Visit www.TM.org

__Set of Weights__

I have two sets of weights at home shown in the picture below.

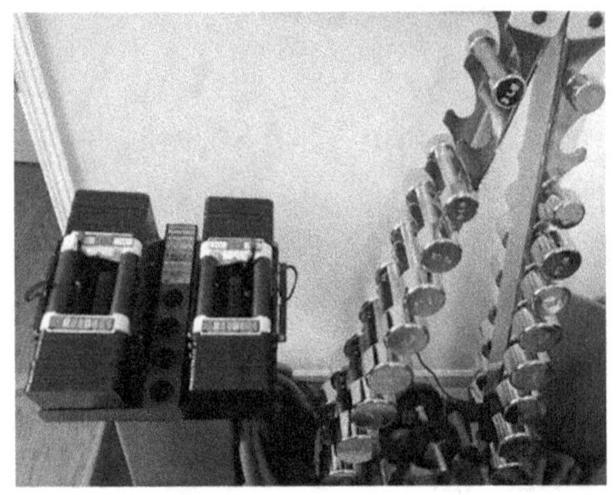

They represent a sizeable investment. When I purchased them over 13 years ago I think the total bill came to $1,500. I consider them one of my most important investments and guess-ti-mate my cost-per-use to be .70¢ – so far. Every day I use them that cost of use goes down further. But cost is not the point for me about these. The value I derive from them has been, and continues to be, enormous.

Over the years I have done yoga daily for an hour a day (a schedule I maintained for several years)...and never really liked it. I made myself swim laps an hour a day, every day, for one whole year...and never really liked it. I have similarly tried bicycling, jogging and other things that – for me – were more tedious than enjoyable. So, if you like or love those things – have at it! Enjoy. Use what works for you!

Some people don't like weightlifting. I love it. I am not a powerlifter; I don't go for the highest weight or the biggest muscles. I weightlift because it helps me drag my sorry butt up rock faces when I rock climb. I know that I will have more fun on the rock because I feel lighter to myself.

__Warm Dead Sea Salt Baths (nearly free, less than $3 per use)__

Once on a rock climbing trip to Santa Barbara, California, I found myself in a health food store looking for Epsom Salts and having trouble finding them. I'd just climbed all day and wanted to take a salt bath, which I knew from experience would minimize my soreness, help me sleep through the night and reduce my overall pain levels.

The store employee told me they only carried this one product from Annie Cunningham's *Dead Sea Warehouse*.[24] I tried it, reluctantly because 5 pounds of this cost about $20 which I thought was too high compared to the Epsom salts I was used to. Boy, was I in for a surprise!

After that first bath I was hooked. Not only did I feel great, I felt *healthier!* This was a quantum level above my old Epsom Salt experience. I went to Annie's website and I found out that Dead Sea Salts have a unique mineral composition that is famous the world over for reducing aches and pains. Now I recommend it to everyone, and each new client I work with is sent home with a free sample and instructions on how to buy more.

Imagine my surprise when I found out that many spas charge as much as $25 a pound for Dead Sea bath salts. I highly recommend regularly taking a warm Dead Sea Salt bath with Annie's product. I also recommend rinsing off with warm water that is slightly cooler than the bath water.

Besides all that, I must share that Annie has become a friend as well as providing me with an important tool that I regularly use. Stay open and experiment. I would never have found this great product or this great friend if I'd not taken a chance and tried it out.

Q-Flex or TheraCane Self Massager

This is another great option for immediate relief. There are several low-tech versions of this self-massage tool on the market. I own three: two Q-Flex and one TheraCane, and have them scattered around my house and office so they're always in easy reach.

---

[24] http://deadseawarehouse.com

The Q-Flex I saw on *Shark Tank*[25] and immediately ordered it. I like it because it fits in my carry-on bag when I travel. It is presented as an acupressure tool which, in my opinion, is a bit more than it is. Sure, it could be used if someone was trained in acupressure, but for the average Joe or Jane, it's just a self-massage tool for getting at knots of tension and helping them unravel a little.

And it works, not nearly as well as the hands of a competent therapist, but for home use or when on the road, I think it's a great Self-Care tool.

My go-to is the TheraCane. It has a longer length and reach which makes it, for me, a more versatile tool. One of my massage therapist friends turned me onto it. She said that during her divorce it was the only thing she and her ex fought over. Ha! I believe it.

I would offer this tip that I follow in using one of these: I use the principle of *Above & Below.* Rather than working directly on the hard or tender spot that may be bothering you, work around it – above and below.

Resist the temptation of finding the exact knot of tension and digging into it with all your might. More pressure is not necessarily better!

Instead, find the tender or knotted spot and then place the tip of the tool slightly above that spot and gently apply pressure there, holding it for a few seconds, and then release it.

Then do the same slightly below the tender spot. If you want, you can also apply a few seconds to the right and to the left of the tender spot.

---

[25] http://abc.go.com/shows/shark-tank

I've found that using the *Above & Below* approach works better than working right on the tender spot.

There are two manufacturers whose products I own.[26]

Gravity Pal® Low Angle Inversion Tables

I believe that inversion should be central to everyone's Wellness plan. I have a passionate mission to assist people who, like myself, have been plagued by chronic back pain. I know how debilitating that can be and my mission is to make Gravity Pal® available to everyone who might derive benefit from it.

I've already presented throughout this book many reasons I hope you'll consider purchasing a Gravity Pal®. Since we're talking about what's in my personal toolkit and why, here's what 1 to 2 minute sessions on my Gravity Pal® does for me:

I receive immediate relief from tension and pain in my back and – as a result of my regular daily use – have experienced a cumulative longer-term relief. This means I am more pain-free for longer periods of time throughout the day, and I also experience whole days and even weeks where I do not experience pain.

Also, I definitely notice my thinking is clearer and my overall sense of vitality and Wellness has improved. For me, more so than any other tool or modality in my toolkit, my Gravity Pal® is the one single tool I would never, ever give up.

Besides that, traveling for me was impossible after a setback I had a few years ago, but now, with my Gravity Pal® *Traveler* and *Checkable Airline Luggage Case* I am good to go. The minute I arrive at my

____

[26] Here are their links: Q-Flex https://getqflex.com and TheraCane
  http://www.theracane.com

destination I set it up and get on it, and in just 1 or 3 minutes I'm ready to move on. I use it whenever and wherever I need.

The More Important Discovery is our
Gravity Pal Inversion Method™

I've already written on this point before but it bears saying again. Our most important discovery is the combination of using the *low* angle for *short* durations of 1 to 3 minutes on a *regular* basis of 2 to 3 times per day. I am amazed by the cumulative effects that people continue to report to me because they use their Gravity Pals regularly.

In the section above I mentioned *Legs Up on the Couch* as an optional free tool. If you're going to do that, then again, I recommend you apply our method the best way you can even though you're not at a low angle and your back is flat. But you can still do it 1 to 3 minutes at a time on a regular basis. I think even that may assist you.

I also think everyone who currently owns a high angle inversion table should consider trying to use it applying the *Gravity Pal Inversion Method™* – using the lowest angle they can. Inversion itself has a value; the *Gravity Pal Inversion Method™*, in my opinion, optimizes that value.

Tools are only valuable when they are used. But the way they are used directly determines the results that people will or will not obtain.

Expensive Investments That May Be Worth It

I mentioned that my weight sets put me back around $1,500 or so about 13 years ago. I checked and the one set, the solid chrome weights, are not being sold anymore and if you can cobble the set together it would cost over $2,000 today. Even my weight blocks cost today about $700, I think I paid less than $500 for them years ago.

Sometimes you luckily find an investment that appreciates in value. But then again, I doubt that I'll be selling them anytime soon. The biggest profit I've received has been the cumulative benefit from using them in my better health and better living.

I've made other much bigger investments in equipment that I'll tell you about in a minute. Before I do, I'll tell you a story about a guy who taught me that before investing in a bigger ticket item I really should look closely at whether I was going to use it.

Actually, this story is not about equipment of any kind and may at first appear to be off-topic – so bear with me for a minute.

Sometimes you learn things from unexpected sources. Sometimes, just in the course of a conversation, a valuable jewel pops out. This story is mostly about why I chose to listen to a random comment a guy made one day that proved to be valuable. The story gives you context why he and I were even talking in the first place.

Dan, the UPS Man

In my little town in Iowa everybody knows Dan, the UPS Man. Always smiling, Dan is the guy the UPS organization should have on its promotional posters and commercials. He's good looking, has a big smile, always has a friendly word, and knows his customers.

One rainy winter day over the lunch hour, my wife and I were leaving a restaurant when we saw SMOKE and FIRE a few doors away. We immediately crossed the street to get out of the way of the crowd that was forming. Dan's UPS truck was parked just across from the fire.

In a flash, *DAN RAN INTO THE BURNING BUILDING!*

We didn't see him come out of the building with a child in his arms, like you might expect from the movies. In fact, we didn't see the rest of the event as the fire department scooted us away from the scene.

But I saw Dan later that day and asked him why he charged into the building like that, and asked what had happened. He told me that he knew an elderly retired lady had an apartment upstairs and said, *"Usually that time of day she's home."*

I thought to myself, *"Only Dan would know that kind of thing!"*

Fortunately, he said, when he got upstairs someone who was exiting the building told him the retired lady was not there that day so he didn't have to rescue her after all.

But to me, Dan was – and is – a hero. Every time I see him I feel proud to know him. His words, still ring in my ears, *"Usually that time of day she's home."*

Dan's Relevant Comment to Me – *"Don't Chase Shiny New Things"*

My conversation with Dan drifted to more mundane things. Dan casually mentioned he was busy with picking up treadmill and other exercise machines that people had purchased as part of their New Year's resolution to exercise more.

He then told me that expensive exercise equipment was the #1 product being returned by customers that month – and that this was the same story every year.

"People chase shiny new things," he said. Maybe it was because the whole day was more emotionally charged, but I took notice and never forgot that comment.

I tell you this story because it points out how I learned to pay attention to *"shiny new things"* when I was in the market to purchase more expensive Self-Care equipment for myself.

When I was really in pain and my tendency was to grab onto the next promise of hope, that little comment from Dan reminded me to slow down and think it through. Dan, "Mr. Credible," taught me a valuable lesson by sharing what he had observed.

Fitness is a nice idea that a lot of people think is cool before they realize they actually have to *do* something. To some degree, Self-Care is like that too.

Except for One Really Important Thing

There are those of us who need to embrace Self-Care and really have to do it. I'm one of them and I wrote this book primarily for those who, like me, can create a significant improvement in their quality of life by merely learning and – most importantly – *doing* a few things on a regular basis.

For us, we can shift from being in a state of chronic pain, discouragement, and fear, to a state of optimism and hope. We *can* accomplish this – I know it firsthand.

Sometimes a really expensive piece of equipment is exactly what may make a difference for us.

What follows are two expensive tools that I own and use. These are not items that most people are going to purchase for themselves. But they are good to know about nonetheless.

Gyrotonic Machine

In 2003 I was still struggling to put together my toolkit. I had discovered a Pilates instructor and my weekly sessions with her were making a difference. Pain levels in my body were decreasing and I began to appreciate the important relationship between keeping the core-abdominal muscles toned and keeping pain levels down.

I had discovered rock climbing, and one of the tools I had recently found to develop grip-strength was a gyroscope-type exercise ball. It was really developing my forearms and I also noticed a new sensation when I did it – my entire arms and shoulders felt what I can only describe as more integrated.

One day I mentioned it to my Pilates instructor and said, *"I wish there was a gyroscope-type device I could use for my whole body."*

To my surprise she said, *"Oh, one exists."* She said she didn't know what it was called but remembered reading about it in one of her trade magazines. So I set out to learn about this cool idea.

What I found was a website, www.Gyrotonic.com. From there I found that, in Iowa, there wasn't at that time a certified trainer, so I had to travel to Chicago to try this out. Fortunately, in 2003 I was doing business in Chicago and regularly traveled there.

Very fortunately, for me, I found a fabulous therapist, Stephanie Davies Devlen O.T., who's also an expert Pilates instructor. I recommend Stephanie as one of the finest therapists I have ever met, and if you are in the Chicago area, please try to see her. Her website is www.sdrehab.com.

Over the next several years I would see Stephanie often. It was clear right away the unique exercises offered using the Gyrotonic machine were making a big difference for me.

So I bought one and followed the routines I learned when back home in Iowa. It was expensive, $6,000, and remains one of the best investments I've ever made. The Gyrotonic machine allows a controlled and weighted "Arch & Curl" type of experience that I need to keep my spine supple; even a few minutes on it is like nothing else for me. I call it my exercise dessert because the feeling I get from using it can only be described as *yummy! :)*

I recommend that you go to their website, find a local certified Gyrotonic instructor and check it out. It may or may not be suitable for your situation, but it's truly one of the most remarkable things I have in my toolkit.

ROM (Range of Motion) Machine

This is the most outrageously expensive item I purchased for myself. It costs as much as a small truck and is only suitable for those who feel they really need it and who actually will use it. Otherwise, it is the king of the shiny new things!

I will tell you it is an awesome piece of equipment. Top, *top shelf.* For me, I had to find something that would help me save maximum time and deliver a quality aerobic workout. Plus I hated the treadmill experience and, try as I might, I could never muster the necessary 30-40 minutes per treadmill session.

With the ROM you get a high quality intensive aerobic workout *in only 4 minutes.* Yes, you read that right – 4 minutes!

My favorite part of working with this machine is its unique 34-inch stair-stepper, with weight resistance. For me, that range of motion exercise has proved to be a blessing.

Between this and my Gyrotonic machine, I'm able to keep my hip girdle open and fluid – a key for managing my own back pain-related issues.

You may have seen the ROM advertisements in flight magazines on airplanes. When I purchased mine in 2006 it cost about $15,000. You can read about it at www.romquickgym.com.

Watch the videos and read the studies they have done on it. I love it, and if you can wrap your head around how much it costs, I highly recommend it.

Special Tools

Both the ROM and Gyrotonic machines are not something most people will ever aspire to own, even though I believe they would potentially serve just about everyone.

They're both unique among Self-Care tools for what they do. They both continue to provide terrific cumulative relief for me, and each are central to my Self-Care toolkit – I love them both. I don't regret purchasing them for a second.

You too may find you need special tools. If you do, I say go ahead and invest in them when it's crystal clear that your life with them can be better than your life without them. You are worth it; finding the right tools is simply a Godsend.

How to Put It All Together – Sustainable Schedules

The final main piece in our toolkit is how we integrate our Modalities and Selected Tools into our lives. Can't we just wing it?

That depends on you; if you're like me, no. For me, I need at least the basic outline of a schedule. I need to know – at least in general – when I'm doing *what* and *next.*

So I have a schedule that I try to keep – emphasis on *try.* Life is full of disruptions, and in order to employ the incredible power of regularity I have to make it simple – otherwise I won't do it.

I find it valuable to keep it as simple as possible and to break it into:

- ❖ Every day, and
- ❖ Every week

Every day, first thing after I'm out of bed, I do the *4 Minute Miracle.* There is a complete presentation on it in the Appendix and I ask you to read about it there but, for now, I'll share these little bits. I wanted something I could do – or approximate – no matter what shape I was in, or what setback or challenge I was facing. I wanted something I could use whether I was coping, improving or celebrating.

This little gem is the result of distilling many years of research and testing. I believe just about everyone can use parts of the *4 Minute Miracle* whether you are young, old, in decent shape or – importantly – in poor shape as well.

I do it standing up, breathing in certain ways while moving in certain ways. Afterward, I spend one minute on a Gravity Pal® enjoying the effects of low angle inversion.

That's it. Super simple, and in four minutes you'll be amazed how much better you'll feel all over your body.

This *4 Minute Miracle:*

- ❖ Stimulates the lymph, activates the brain, and relaxes the tissues all over your body
- ❖ Expands your lung capacity and strengthens your immune system,
- ❖ Increases your physical endurance and your ability to walk upstairs while keeping your breath
- ❖ As a special bonus, it will dramatically improve the tone of your core abdominal muscles – including your pelvic floor and your lower back muscles

You can do the *4 Minute Miracle* in your socks, in your living room or anywhere

– and it only takes 4 minutes

As mentioned above, there's a complete presentation on the *4 Minute Miracle* in the Appendix which I give to you, dear reader, for free. Please use it; it's wonderful. On my website, www.GravityPal. com, we offer for sale a handy booklet on the *4 Minute Miracle* which includes a video. I humbly believe it's an awesome tool, and besides developing Gravity Pal® and the *Gravity Pal Inversion Method™* it's the thing I am most proud and happy to share with you and the world.

So, every day, the first thing I do is the *4 Minute Miracle* which includes 1 or 2 minutes on my Gravity Pal®. It always amazes me how better my day starts with this few minute routine.

Every evening, just before going to bed, I also spend 1 to 3 minutes on my Gravity Pal®. Plus, I usually have one or two more 1 to 3 minute Gravity Pal® sessions throughout the day as I think of it or feel the need for it.

Those are the only things I always do every day. Besides that, I try to find time to walk every day and that includes taking "the long way around" while out and about.

My Weekly Schedule is a Rough Outline

I fit in various things I need to do to maintain my Wellness schedule. On paper it looks like this:

Sunday: Weights (2/3 intensity) and aerobic workout at home

Monday: Massage from my massage therapist

Tuesday: ROM for 4 minutes & Gyrotonic Session

Wednesday: Weights (full intensity) and aerobic workout with
                my fitness trainer + Salt Bath

Thursday: ROM for 4 minutes & Zero Balancing session
                I receive from my wife, Dawn

Friday: Weights (1/3 intensity) and aerobic workout at home

Saturday: ROM for 4 minutes & day off – but I often do yard work
                that day

I also have to fit in a Chiropractic and Acupuncture session about once every month or two. So, sketch it out. It helps to write it down or put it in your electronic schedule. Make it work for you.

Here are a few more tips about setting up your schedule:

1. Keep it simple and as minimal as possible – **but do something EVERY DAY**

2. Add new things to do one at a time

3. Pay attention to what works, and keep doing it

4. Keep it fresh – once it's boring or not fun,
    add something to it or find something else to do

5. Keep looking, and keep experimenting

Making it Real

Self-Care is an assemblage of many tools, all of which have to mesh with one's personality and lifestyle; otherwise they will only be nice ideas. The real work is making them fit into our lives.

There's an old saying, *"The knowledge in the book remains in the book."* All the wisdom in books is absolutely worthless as long as it only exists in the book. We have to read it, appreciate it, and apply it. Knowledge must be put into action; all the fruits are found in the field of action.

I've emphasized that Self-Care is about *doing* because I've found that the fruits come from what we do regularly. That power of regularity is one of the biggest secrets of Self-Care.

If you take two things from this book, I hope they will be these two things:

1. Do something every day

2. Commit to a minimum time every day – even only 2 or 3 minutes. If you can stretch that into 15 or more minutes – all the better! But make sure you do your 2-3 minutes *every day.*

The two words "short duration" are important simply because if you start something every day, you will, at very least, keep the daily habit.

Comedian Jerry Seinfeld in an interview said that in his earliest days he developed the habit of writing every day for at least 30 minutes. Some days those 30 minutes spilled over into hours of inspired material, and some days those 30 minutes were a painful eternity. His progress came out of his long-term commitment to always do *something.* Every. Day. Regularly.

Be Like Jerry

Committing to a few minutes of Self-Care every day sets the stage for you to experience *cumulative* results. It's amazing the transformation that we can create for ourselves by merely embracing those two concepts:

* *Short-duration*
* *Regular daily experience*

The world tears at our attention to run after the next new shiny thing. We will be endlessly tempted to drop our routine and selected tools. There's nothing wrong with taking on new additional tools, provided you can make the next new thing also fit into your busy days. Don't get distracted. You're shooting for cumulative results.

Here are two tips to make it even simpler and easier:

1. **Pick one thing to do every day for 2 to 4 minutes, and do it for 90 days**. Heck, it's only going to take 2 to 4 minutes!

2. **Pick a time and keep it**. This is what I do – first thing in the morning I do the *4 Minute Miracle,* and last thing before bed I spend 2-3 minutes on my Gravity Pal®.

The easiest thing of all is if your selected tools and modalities are self-reinforcing (because you enjoy and derive such benefit from them). When I designed the Gravity Pal® I wanted it to be so effective that users would effortlessly add it to their daily routine.

Based on the feedback we receive, it appears this is exactly what people experience. It's easy to see cumulative results when it's self-reinforcing to experience.

It's no secret Gravity Pal® is my go-to tool and I believe it may be appropriate for most of you as well. But I never lose sight of the fact that it is only one tool. The most important thing for your Self-Care program is to create a toolkit you can use regularly that delivers the cumulative results you need – whether that includes Gravity Pal® or not.

You're On a New Journey

When you embrace the *Four Dance Steps of Wellness,* when you're deep in the *coping* stage, you're starting a new path that offers incredible growth and opportunities to learn. The #1 biggest thing you'll learn will be about your own self. Just by keeping focused on doing something to address your health and Wellness on a daily basis, insights about *you* will come into focus.

And it is all for the good. You'll definitely find out how you resist things and how you, in fact, may be your own worst enemy. And if that's the case – ain't that great!?! Why?

Because You've Elevated that "Resisted-Thing" to a Choice!

❖ So you find out you have a habit of procrastinating – well, *now* that's a choice!

❖ You've discovered you have a habit of discouraging self-talk – *now* that's a new choice!

I quickly found out that I'm great at making a schedule but I resist following it when I'm not in pain. Well, guess what? It didn't take long to discover that I would backslide! No surprises there. But I had to elevate this new knowing about myself to a choice and here is the biggest lesson of all:

Every Moment is a New Choice

Embracing this truth has had many broad impacts on my life. I am more empowered in a whole host of ways because I've embraced this idea. In many ways I now look at my whole life as being blessed because of my circumstances and the challenges I've had to face.

Sure, sometimes, I wish I didn't have to focus on my toolkit so much. Sure, a part of me wishes that I was like that guy I met at the lunch counter who said he had never experienced any pain – ever!

That's just natural. In fact, I accept it as the nature of being human to always want more and to always imagine – and desire – another way we can be even happier than we already are.

You're Part of a Self-Care Revolution that's Beginning to Sweep the World

If you can imagine, by being in less pain and being willing to work at it, you're part of something momentous. As you already know, Self-Care is *not* Alone-Care. We need our *team.* We need each other.

By simply shifting your role in your own health and Wellness process to that of team leader and General Contractor, you'll impact everyone else in your team and everyone who knows you or hears about you. Your own Self-Care process will not only help you but will inspire others to follow your example.

And as the numbers of people embracing Self-Care expand all around us, I believe we can all live better.

CHAPTER 10

THE SELF-CARE REVOLUTION IS JUST STARTING

Why Now?

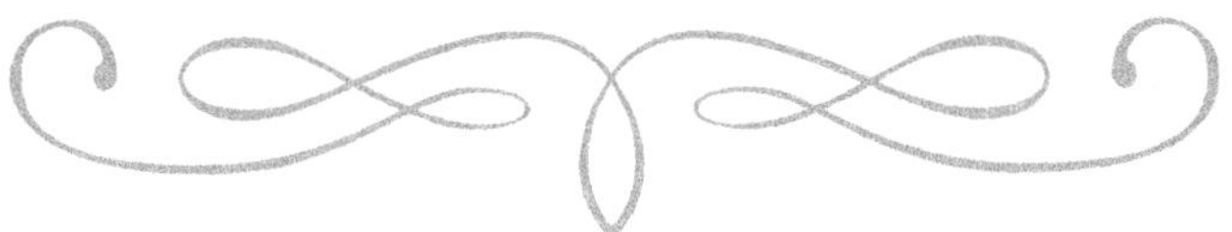

It is an AWESOME time to be alive.

Never before in human history have we had such potential – each and every one of us – to live life in greater ease and comfort while we choose to learn anything we want to learn or to enjoy our leisure time in an array of ways simply unimaginable only a few years ago.

Of course, I can hear those who are thinking, *"What about all the challenges of our time?"* Certainly, we cannot ignore them. There are many surrounding us from all sides. It's our choice of what we want to focus on.

But that's the point: we have more choices than ever before to focus on. And we're living a lot longer while we think about all the many choices we now have.

Increasingly our Biggest Challenge is our Good Fortune

We're living longer – and likely to live even longer still. Breakthroughs are happening every day that promise longer and longer lifespans. Better information options allow us to become more educated about these breakthroughs than ever before.[27]

However, we don't just want to just live longer; we want to enjoy our longer lives and NOT live in a long, miserable decline in health.

People Want to Live Longer – But Pain Free & Vibrantly

Up until about 1750 there was very little technological progress in human society. You could expect very little innovation or

---

[27] I recommend everyone subscribe to the free service offered by *Medical News Today*, http://www.medicalnewstoday.com

improvement in any field during your lifetime. Whether it was transportation, communication, food storage options, hygiene, basic comforts or health care tools, like inversion methods for example, there was tremendous similarity of life in 1750 with those who had lived 1,000 or 2,000 years before. You could expect the conditions of life and the technologies that could make life easier not to change much for you – or your children or your grandchildren.

No more. *The times they are a-changin' – and fast.* Today we expect life to be radically different *continuously.* We can barely forecast the changes coming at us in the next few years!

And while we are experiencing continuous radical change, our lifespans are getting longer and longer. In 2006, Barron's Magazine had an entire issue devoted to advances in longevity, its front page had the provocative title, *"Live to Be 150. There's a person alive who'll live to be over 150 – and they are 60 years old today."* [28]

That may be overly optimistic but it's a safe bet advances in longevity will be profound in the coming years. We don't know if our lives may be extended 5, 10, 50 years – or longer. Those of us who deal with chronic pain know we don't want longer years while in pain. We want relief and we want it *now.*

We can certainly hope there'll be advances that eliminate chronic pain. But the only thing we can be certain of, and the only thing we have control over is what we choose to do today. My dear friend and chiropractor, Dr. Charles Coram, brilliantly sums it up this way, *"We have to start something or stop something."* We must become proactive about our Self-Care.

---

[28] Palmer, Jay. "Live to 150." Barron's. April 17, 2006. Accessed April 26, 2017.
   http://www.barrons.com/articles/SB114506274084226747

This is Both Good News and *Challenging* News

Today, the biggest challenge is adapting to change. Change, and the challenge of adapting to it, is not going away. For many, this can be very stressful, particularly when we recognize we may need to economically support ourselves for many years longer than we had ever planned for – or anyone in human history ever thought was possible.

The challenge is good but the stress is not. Here's the difference between *challenge* and *stress.*

Dr. Fred Travis in his excellent book, *Your Brain is a River Not a Rock,* points out the important distinction between being stressed and challenged.

"We need to distinguish between stress and challenge. Some people say that they need "stress" to function at their best, that under "stress" they are more creative. They are probably talking about the enhancing effects of <u>challenge</u> rather than the debilitating effects of <u>stress</u>.

*"Under challenge, we are required to think and act at our upper limits of abilities. **Challenge supports optimal performance.***

"But when the challenge gets too high and we feel that we cannot succeed, the brain downshifts into a stress response.

"People … perform at optimal levels if they are challenged, and perform at reduced levels if they are stressed." [29]

---

[29] Travis, Frederick, Ph.D., *Your Brain is a River Not a Rock,*
ISBN-13: 978-1469937212, pp. 185-186

Self-Care is a challenge. The trick is not to let it become a stress.
Self-Care requires we act in a manageable, step by step *process.*
We must find tools that effectively reduce stress and use them.

Facing the Challenge with Self-Care

The real challenge of our time is to recognize that Self-Care is not an option. More and more people are coming to this realization. They need direction, strategies, resources and tools that work for them.

And they need inspiration. There's a great book I recommend, especially to younger people, titled *"Growing Old is Not for Sissies."* [30] It's a series of portraits of senior athletes and is quite inspiring. I came across this book when I turned 40 and it made a big impression on me.

Imagining our life far beyond 100 years – in vibrant good health – is not only possible but increasingly likely. Robert Marchand, the French amateur cyclist is more aerobically fit at the age of 105 than most 50-year-olds, and appears to be getting even fitter as he ages. He is the focus of a new study of his physiology which appeared in the December 2016 issue of *The Journal of Applied Physiology.*[31]

And while it is true that Mr. Marchand is – as of right now – an exceptional "outlier," he is pointing the way to where we are all headed ...

... if we choose to be...

---

[30] Clark, Etta, *Growing Old is Not for Sissies*, Pomegranate, August 1986
http://www.ettaclark.com

[31] *Lessons on Aging Well, From a 105-Year-Old Cyclist,* https://www.nytimes.com/2017/02/08/well/move/lessons-on-aging-well-from-a-105-year-old-cyclist.html?_r=0, accessed April 25, 2017

We can choose to emulate Mr. Marchand the best way we can. Or we can simply look at how complex our healthcare system has become and how crazy expensive everything is – and despair.

Certainly, we can choose to simply ride it out, not take charge and let the healthcare system try its best to provide us what we need. That too is a choice.

The New Self-Care Paradigm

But if you've read this book I'm betting you're interested in taking more control over your healthcare *process.* In that case you're not simply going to submit to the healthcare system but are going to become an active and central participant to your own healthcare.

This new process is <u>not</u> Alone-Care.

This new process is about your involvement; it's about building teams, developing your Self-Care toolkit and becoming the General Contractor of your own healthcare.

This new process is beyond general fitness and beyond the simple idea of prevention.

The New Focus is on Balance and Regaining Balance

We learned in Chapter 5 in our discussion on the *Six Stages of Disease* that no matter how hard we try to maintain balance in the human physiology, life itself is going to cause imbalances – big and small – with which we will constantly have to contend.

Because we know this, keeping our focus on harnessing the body's natural tendency to restore balance becomes our core prevention and maintenance principle.

Self-Care will always be a choice. Some will jump right on it today. Many of you already have. Others will put this book down and let it collect dust.

Remember this: the knowledge in the book remains in the book.

The really good news is that every moment offers us a new choice.

Self-Care starts when you decide.

APPENDIX

I. **Supplemental Bonuses to Chapter 9 on Building Your Toolkit**

    a. The 4 Minute Miracle
    b. Drinking Water as a Key to Pain Management & Wellness
    c. The *Gravity Pal Inversion Method™*

II. **Resource Guide**

    a. Modalities I Regularly Use and Recommend
    b. Useful Websites & Books
    c. Tools I Have Found Useful

III. **An Invitation to Researchers**

I. Supplemental Information to Chapter 9 on Building Your Toolkit

This section provides additional information regarding the *4 Minute Miracle* and on *Drinking Water as a Key to Pain Management & Wellness*.

a. The 4 Minute Miracle

No matter what shape you're in – you can still breathe. And as long as you have control over breathing you can exercise. Breathing in combination with small movements can be powerful exercises that virtually everyone, regardless of fitness level, can perform.

My ongoing desire in developing this exercise routine was to reduce pain in my body and – simultaneously – keep my abs toned, kick start my brain aerobically, stimulate my lymph system, and decompress my spine – all in 5 minutes or less.

What follows is a series of short exercises I developed for myself and for people who have compression related pain issues, or simply want to add an invigorating wake-up to their day. It is also great for those who are afraid to start exercising because they think they're not in good enough shape or don't have any idea where to start.

This *4 Minute Miracle* is a great place to start.

I also recommend this series as a way to leverage time – meaning to get the most out of the least time spent. For me, it's a flat-out miracle how much benefit I derive from this little 4 minute routine. I think if you do this daily for 3 months, you too will be tremendously impressed.

Over the course of several months you may also notice many side-benefits to this series besides improved spinal decompression. These would include strengthening of the lower back muscles, toning of the core and ab muscles, improved lung capacity and brain boost, stimulation to the lymph system (which also serves your internal organs), as well as improvements in your energy levels, digestion, and overall circulation.

This series is not a replacement for regular full sessions of other exercise programs whether you like yoga, Pilates or aerobics. Please continue other exercise programs you enjoy. The *4 Minute Miracle* was not designed to be a total body only-thing-you-need kind of exercise series. It's a way to "prime the pump" and start the day, and for me it's a way to make sure I get the best start possible.

My Morning Exercises were
Reducing Pain in My Body ... *but ...*

Previous to developing the *4 Minute Miracle* I was spending upwards of 30 minutes each morning doing an array of exercises that, happily, reduced pain for me. The reduced pain was great and needed, but too many days I just couldn't fit in the time, and those days were more painful. I needed something that would take less time I could do *every day* that would make a difference.

After many years of trial and error I finally figured it out.

The *4 Minute Miracle* is an amalgam of specific exercises I've discovered and used over many years. These include influences from yoga[32], Pilates[33], Gyrokenesis[34] and BrainGym.[35] The initial inspiration came from strongman Matt Furey's standing ab exercises, a person to whom I'm particularly grateful.[36]

For average people or those in marginal or even poor health, a little of the *4 Minute Miracle* can go a long way. I believe that almost everyone can do them – or approximate them.

Of course, please consult your doctor or primary health care provider before starting this or any new exercise or activity.

---

[32] To find a credentialed yoga teacher I recommend starting here, https://www.yogaalliance.org/Directory

[33] https://en.wikipedia.org/wiki/Pilates, For instructors, https://www.pilates.com/BBAPP/V/education/instructor-directory.html

[34] https://wwww.gyrotonic.com/about/gyrokinesis-method

[35] http://www.braingym.org

[36] For an Ab Workout suitable for advanced athletes please see *Combat Abs*, by Matt Furey, http://www.mattfurey.com

Getting Started

The *4 Minute Miracle* is the very first thing I do in the morning after splashing water on my face. The way I do it takes a total of about 4 minutes including a minute on my Gravity Pal®. They'll take you a few minutes more while you're learning but it won't take you long to master them.

There is nothing magical about the 4 minutes, per se. I limit the time for two reasons: in the morning I want to get going right away and, therefore, spend the least amount of time to do anything!

The second reason is because I know myself, and if I had to set aside more time for this I would simply not do it as regularly. If you have the time and inclination to expand the time commitment, have at it!

But, again, I default to what I know I can do regularly that gets me the results I am looking for. This series complements all the other ways I like to exercise and, I believe, will do the same for you.

I have provided below a description of each of the *4 Minute Miracle* exercises.

Please Note: There are two considerations before you get started:

First, as with any exercise program, make sure that you are at least approximately fit to do these exercises. My bet is that most people will have no problem with them. However, prudence dictates that you should consult your physician or primary health care provider before starting the *4 Minute Miracle* for two reasons:

1. The biggest reason, in my opinion, is that your physician or primary health care provider are on your Self-Care team. You should get in the habit of telling your team members what

you are both doing and what you're evaluating. This is a great place for you to start that habit.

2. The more obvious reason is that you may have some health consideration where it is important for you to avoid – *or modify in some way* – these exercises. I cannot know this for every person reading this in spite of my enthusiastic belief that these exercises are probably okay for just about everyone. Again, this is a clear example when you should use your team members as collaborators in your Self-Care process.

The second consideration: what follows is an outline of the exercises. It will get you started. If you want more detail please watch the video demonstration available at www.GravityPal.com. After you try it for a few weeks I hope you'll want to share the *4 Minute Miracle* with your friends.

Exercises of the *4 Minute Miracle*

1. Almost Whistling
2. The Vacuum
3. The Curling Over & Arching Up
4. Side Bend, Pump & Crunch Stretches – Two Ways (do both)
5. Standing Pump Crunches
6. Marching Cross Knee Slappers

These six short exercises are followed by one minute on a Gravity Pal® or another inversion table set to its lowest setting. Alternatively, use *Legs on the Couch* outlined in Chapter 9.

Tips

1. Each exercise is done standing with toes pointed forward
2. You always breathe _in_ through your nose and _out_ through your mouth
3. Do all of these on an empty stomach
4. Start with one repetition. Add reps slowly. You may never choose to go over 3 or 4 reps, and that's okay
5. If you feel light-headed, stop, rest, and restart. This can happen when you start these exercises, but very soon your body will get used to having more oxygen in it

<u>Almost Whistling</u>

Tip: *you can also do this sitting at a red light in your car*

- ❖ Stand with Both Feet Shoulder-Width Apart

- ❖ Breathe Deeply in Through Your Nose Filling Your Upper Lungs

- ❖ Pause for One Second

- ❖ Through a Teeny Little Opening Between Your Teeth Slowly Let Out a Tiny Stream of Air – Will Sound Almost Like a Whistle – sssss – Until You're Out of Breath

- ❖ When All Your Breath is Out Suck In Your Gut and Hold It for a Few Seconds

- ❖ Breathe in Deeply Through Your Nose – and Start Again

- ❖ Repeat 2 to 4 Times

<u>The Vacuum</u>

Holding your breath out while holding your gut in

- ❖ Stand with Both Feet Shoulder-Width Apart

- ❖ Breathe Deeply in Through Your Nose Filling Your Upper Lungs

- ❖ Pause for One Second

- ❖ Exhale in a Great Whoosh Out Your Mouth While at the Same Time Bending Over Forward as Far as It's Comfortable

- ❖ While Bent Over, Try to Squeeze Out the Last Ounces of Breath and When You've Reached Your Limit, Press Your Tongue Up Onto the Roof of Your Mouth

- ❖ Come Up to Standing Halfway Erect, Lift the Diaphragm and <u>Hold Your Position</u> Not Letting ANY Air In For 5 to 7 Seconds

- ❖ Let Go and Breathe In and Out Normally For a Few Breaths

- ❖ Relax For a Second

- ❖ Breathe Deeply in Through Your Nose, Filling Your Upper Lungs and Start Again

- ❖ <u>PLEASE NOTE:</u> When you first try this you may feel out of breath after the first repetition. Don't worry. This will pass as you continue to do this exercise daily.

- ❖ Repeat 2 to 4 Times

At first you may not feel a connection with your Ab Muscles. Don't worry. It won't take long before you'll connect with your deeper muscles and suck in your gut to an amazing degree. This exercise is, in my opinion, one of the most important as it strengthens the diaphragm and – very importantly for both men and women – the pelvic floor.

The Curling Over & Arching Up
Like doing a slow curling sit-up – only you're standing

Followed by arching your back – like a Cobra yoga pose – only you're standing

❖ **Stand with Both Feet Shoulder-Width Apart**

❖ **Breathe Deeply in Through Your Nose, Filling Your Upper Lungs**

❖ **Pause for One Second**

❖ **Exhale a Small Channel of Air While Slowly Curling Over Following Your Chin to a Fully Bent Over Position**

❖ **TIP: It's as if you're scraping the front of your chest with your chin while squeezing all of the air out of your body**

❖ **While You're Doing This Connect With Your Abs as if You're Curling Over Them**

❖ **When You're at the Bottom of Curling Over, SLOWLY Arch Your Back Until You're Standing Straight Up**

❖ **Repeat 2 to 4 times**

- ❖ After You've Done 2 to 4 Reps, Do One Rep at a 45 Degree Angle to the Left and then One Rep at a 45 Degree Angle to the Right

- ❖ Repeat Those 45 Degree Angle Reps 2 to 4 times

Side Bend, Pump & Crunch Stretches – Two Ways (do both)
Super easy, good morning stretches

First Way – One Hand Reaching Up and One Hand Reaching Down

- ❖ Stand with Both Feet Shoulder-Width Apart

- ❖ Breathe Deeply in Through Your Nose, Filling Your Upper Lungs

- ❖ Pause for One Second

- ❖ Reach Right Hand Straight Up So Your Arm Almost Touches Your Ear

- ❖ Reach Left Hand Straight Down So Your Hand is Touching Outside of Left Leg

- ❖ Lean to Left

- ❖ Pump Right Hand Up in Rhythm with Short Out-Breaths while Crunching Abs

** and at the same time **

- ❖ Pump Left Hand Down in Rhythm with Short Out-Breaths while Crunching Abs

❖ Breathe in, Reverse and Repeat: Reaching Left Hand Up and Right Hand Down

❖ Do Once (or more if you like) On Each Side

Second Way – _Both Hands Reaching Up Overhead Together with Fingers Interlocked_

❖ Stand with Both Feet Shoulder-Width Apart

❖ Breathe Deeply in Through Your Nose, Filling Your Upper Lungs

❖ Pause for One Second

❖ Interlock Fingers of Both Hands and Reach Way Up Above Your Head

❖ Lean to the Right, Stretch and PAUSE for One Second

❖ Pump & Crunch Abs in Rhythm with Out-Breath Until You're All Out of Breath

❖ Breathe In Again Through Your Nose, Filling Up Upper Lungs

❖ Lean to the Left, Stretch and PAUSE for One Second

❖ Pump & Crunch Abs in Rhythm with Out-Breath Until You're All Out of Breath

❖ Do Once (or more if you like) On Each Side

<u>Standing Pump Crunches</u>

*Try to make you belly button touch your spine at a 45° upward angle –
and try not to laugh – ha!*

❖ **Stand with Both Feet Shoulder-Width Apart**

❖ **Breathe Deeply in Through Your Nose, Filling Your Upper
Lungs**

❖ **Pause for One Second**

❖ **Like You're Blowing Out a Candle, Let Air Out Your Mouth
in Teeny Quick Exhales While Pulling <u>In</u> Your Abs in Rhythm
With Each Exhale.**

   **TIP: Imagine Your Belly Button is Trying to Reach Upward and
   Touch a Spot in the Middle of Your Upper Back Between Your
   Shoulder Blades – With Each Exhale**

❖ **Try To Do 10 or More Exhales Before You Run Out of Breath**

❖ **When You're Out of Breath: Pause & Pull in Your Abs and
Hold Them in Tight for Several Seconds**

❖ **Do This Twice**

<u>Marching Cross Knee Slappers</u>

These Cross-Crawls are inspired by Braingym.com – Check them out

*This exercise is great for your brain, upper legs,
hips and lower abs – all at the same time*

❖ Stand with Both Feet Shoulder-Width Apart

❖ Breathe Deeply in Through Your Nose, Filling Your Upper Lungs

❖ Pause for One Second

❖ As if Marching in a Band, Lift Your LEFT Leg Up and When Your Thigh is as High as You Can Manage Slap Your LEFT Thigh Lightly With Your RIGHT Hand

❖ Alternate Between Legs As You Keep Marching and Slapping in Place

❖ Repeat for a Total of 4 to 10 Slaps on Each Thigh

***End Session: One Minute on Gravity Pal® Low Angle
Inversion Table***

Follow these exercises by immediately getting on your Gravity Pal® low angle inversion table for 1 minute.

After you exit your Gravity Pal®, rest comfortably on the floor for 15 to 30 seconds before getting up. I like to use a pillow for this rest period.

Impacts of the 4 Minute Miracle

While developing this exercise series, I was looking for several things that – all together – would support my back health, reduce pain in my body, and assist my overall health. These were:

- ❖ Abdominal Muscle Toning & Back Strengthening
- ❖ Improved Lung Capacity & a Morning Aerobic Brain Boost
- ❖ Stimulation of the Lymph System & Internal Organs
- ❖ Improved Energy, Digestion, and Overall Circulation
- ❖ Spinal Decompression

Abdominal Muscle Toning & Back Strengthening

If I had to pick one group of muscles you need to keep toned I would pick the core muscles which, by my definition, includes everything from your knee caps to your armpits.

Your core muscles are more than just your Ab Muscles. It's a mistake to think that Ab Muscles <u>alone</u> need to be developed.

This series will start the toning of your core and Ab Muscles with a minimal amount of time and effort. You're never going to get a six-pack with them, and they're no substitute for a more dedicated focus on core and abdominal muscle development as you can obtain from Pilates, in particular.

But this series will have a positive impact on all your core and ab muscles. These include the Rectus Abdominis, Internal & External Obliques, Transverse Abs, Quadratus Lumborum, Psoas, Diaphragm and others – all of which are important for back health and back pain relief.

How long will it take for you to notice any effects? That depends on where you're at when you start, but my experience is that you'll start noticing effects right away, and within a few months you'll be looking and feeling much better.

Good core and Ab Muscle tonality helps maintain your back health. ***Too much weight in the belly?* It's pulling on your back muscles and spine.**

Getting rid of belly weight is a different conversation. Belly fat may be due to the visceral fat you've stored in between and around your organs. Removing that fat is a different matter that would likely require adjustments to your diet in combination with exercise. But don't let that fact discourage you.

You need some basic tone in your belly muscles to keep lower back pain under control. This will help.

Lung Capacity & A Morning Aerobic Brain Boost

The deep inhalations into your upper lungs during these exercises will expand your lung capacity and, in combination with ending the session with a minute of low angle inversion, delivers oxygen all over the body, including the brain.

In a remarkably short period of time you'll notice that you're not out of breath when you climb stairs or do anything aerobic. You're also likely to notice that your brain is more awake and lively.

Trust me, even a little of this exercise series followed by a minute of low angle inversion goes a long way.

Stimulation of the Lymph System & Internal Organs

The entire lymphatic system is stimulated and hundreds of lymph nodes will be activated to digest larger molecules of waste material coming their way.

This is particularly significant in the brain where, in 2015, researchers at the University of Virginia identified – for the first time in medical history – lymph vessels in the upper cranium servicing the brain. We address this important finding more in our *Invitation to Researchers* later in this Appendix.

It is interesting to note that old-time body builders were not only focused on the core and Ab Muscles for surface and deep level strength. They believed that developing and keeping toned the these muscles would both protect the internal organs *and strengthen their functioning.*

I'm not aware of any scientific research – yet – that supports that notion, but I believe there's a connection between improved conditioning of these muscles and improved functioning of the internal organs.

This is my working theory:

The combination of deep breathing and small, focused Ab Muscle movements of the *4 Minute Miracle* – when followed by even one minute of low angle inversion – *stimulates the functioning and potentially even the strength of internal belly organs both individually as well as the functions between them.*

I would love to see objective scientific research in this important area.

Improved Energy, Digestion, and Overall Circulation

Breathing deeply, bringing more oxygen into the body, moving the body, and stimulating the circulation of blood, lymph, and cerebrospinal fluid has proven to be a very good way for me to start the day. Its effects carry over beyond the few minutes I invest in the *4 Minute Miracle* and benefit me in many ways.

My energy levels and digestion have improved by my regular daily practice of this simple routine. I was not looking for these effects, but am happy to receive them.

In addition, and perhaps most importantly, I consistently notice that any pain levels in my body significantly drop off after these exercises. I believe the combination of the specific exercise movements, the specific breathing, and the time on my Gravity Pal® all contribute and help me start the day with less pain.

Again, I would like to invite researchers to look more closely at this to objectively evaluate these reported results.[37]

---

[37] One study found improvements in skeletal muscle pain syndrome from regular yoga sessions compared with a control group. Even though this study was focused on yoga movement and breathing exercises, I include this study here as a reference point for researchers who may be interested in studying the effects of exercises that combine specific movement and specific breathing methods, like yoga.

Effects of yoga exercise on maximum oxygen uptake, cortisol level, and creatine kinase myocardial bond activity in female patients with skeletal muscle pain syndrome, Journal of Physical Therapy Science, Min-Sung Ha, et al, May 2015, https://www.ncbi.nlm.nih.gov/pmc/articles/PMC4483416

This study concluded, "*Regular and continuous aerobic exercise such as yoga improves body composition, maximum oxygen uptake, cortisol level, and creatine kinase myocardial bond activity in female patients with skeletal muscle pain syndrome.*"

Spinal Decompression

Most of this comes from the one minute on the Gravity Pal®, but some comes from the various exercises in the series. The cumulative spinal decompression effects I've experienced from even one minute on a Gravity Pal®, experienced every day, are truly astounding. My favorite part of the *4 Minute Miracle* is the final minute I spend on my Gravity Pal®.

Please go to www.GravityPal.com to learn more about the *4 Minute Miracle.*

b. Drinking Water as a Key to Pain Management & Wellness

I listed this as the most essential of the Free Stuff in your toolkit for two reasons:

1) Even though water is vital to our bodily functions, how much water we should drink is a surprisingly controversial subject, and

2) The right level of hydration – which means a proper balance of water functioning in our body – is directly relevant to the conversation of pain and pain relief. Notice I used the word "functioning." Water has a function in the body and we need to appreciate the many ways it is relevant to both pain management and overall health.

The body needs water like a car needs oil – but it is even more essential than that. Seventy-five percent of the body *is water.*

All functions: breathing, thinking, nerve conduction, muscle movement, digestion and more – all require water to work. Every cell, joint, muscle, brain cell and nerve fiber needs water, complains when it's thirsty, and is compromised if not enough water is there.

I refer to our bodies' combination of fibers and fluids as our *"wet gooey stuff."* Some of our stuff is more liquid-wet, and some more solid-wet. But the overall environment is really wet and gooey.

Our Cells Can Dry Out and
Our *"Wet Gooey Stuff"* Becomes More Sticky

Muscularly, a stickier cellular environment allows tight spots and adhesions to more easily form and develop into a source of pain in the body.

Even worse, more sticky muscle tissue makes it much harder to get rid of muscular tight spots and adhesions. As a massage therapist I know that I can smooth out adhesions all day long but if the cells need more moisture, those adhesions are going to either barely release, or simply stay put.

The discs in your spine are like thick sponges. If they're allowed to dry out, this *directly* impacts the health of your spine. Not good.

As mentioned above, the whole body is about 75% water. However, different areas of the body are made up of more or less water; the bones, for example, are about 20% water, whereas the blood is almost 85% water. Your muscles, brain and nervous system are all about 75% water.

Dehydration Causes Systemic
Interaction Problems Within the Body

For example, when hydration levels fall, proper signaling between nerves are interrupted, which causes muscles to function poorly.

If you're in pain it's incredibly important to have the right balance of water in your body. Please notice, I said, *"right balance."* Don't go out and try to flood the body with water. That too, is not good.

Having the right balance of water in your cells allows massage and manipulation techniques (like chiropractic) to be more effective. It allows sessions on a Gravity Pal® to be more effective. When properly hydrated, all systems in the body operate better:

- ❖ **Tissues can move and are more pliable.** This allows important shifts from tension to greater relaxation of tissues.
- ❖ **Cells can absorb nutrients efficiently.** This provides a better environment for cellular health.
- ❖ **Cells can better eliminate waste.** This is a BIGGIE. Cells that are too dry are an invitation to problems. Recall that the first stage of disease is imbalance in the body. Cells that are too dry are like neon lights shouting, *"Relocate here! This is a great place for problems to manifest!"*
- ❖ **Systemic interactions – all systemic interactions throughout the body – operate optimally in an environment of balanced hydration**

People who don't drink enough water are prime targets for pain and other problems caused by dehydration.

Will Drinking More Water *Cure* My Pain?

Maybe, but not probably. This is one point in the controversy. There are those who have made specious claims of having cured a number of diseases simply by drinking water. While it's true that insufficient water balance in the body can be a source of many problems it's a mistake, in my opinion, to jump to the idea that simply drinking more water may cure a disease.

But drinking the right balance water for you can help – a lot. It is possible that in your case, all you need is to increase the amount of water you're drinking and your pain may go away – there are reports that this has happened. But in most cases, saying water can cure pain is a gross overstatement which I think is simply false, and distracts us from the more important conversation about water and how it can help us reduce and manage pain in our lives.

So let's start with one truth that is beyond debate: drinking and maintaining the right *balance* of water – **and most importantly *absorbing* that water** – is essential for everyone to not only maintain good health, but also to keep pain levels to a minimum.

A Practical Way to Discover: *How Much Water Do I Need?*

It depends on many factors. Let's take a minute to discuss how much you may need.

On one end of the spectrum, you'll find people who'll insist you must drink a specific amount of water daily. Often you'll see a formula telling you to drink an additional ½ ounce of water for every pound of your body weight. Weigh 200 pounds? They say to drink an additional 100 ounces of water every day.

On the other end, you'll find those who say to just add a few glasses of water per day and you'll be fine. Who's right?

First, here's a fact that's true for everyone: **YOU MUST REPLACE WHAT YOU USE EVERY DAY**.

If you don't replace what you use, your joints and all your cells and tissues will dry out and every function in the body will try to adjust to that more-dry condition. Your "wet gooey stuff" will become more dense and this will impact all of your cells and all of your bodily functions.

If you continue to shortchange your body the water you're using up every day, over time the more dry the whole body will get, and you can add layer upon layer of imbalance – and problems.

How Much Water Do You Use Up Every Day?

This depends on your body size, activity levels and whether it's particularly hot or cold outside.

On average, our daily bodily functions use up about 60 ounces of water per day and as much as 100+ ounces per day.

Every day we use up on average:

- ❖ Breathing   12 oz
- ❖ Skin Evaporation   12 oz (yes, your skin breathes too!)
- ❖ Urination   26 oz
- ❖ Bowel Movements   6 oz
- ❖ Sweating   4 oz with little activity <u>but</u> over 40 oz (or more) for one hour of exercise

Here's the good news: We can get water from many sources other than drinking glasses of it. Pure drinking water is the best source for your water intake. However, your body can *extract* water from the various beverages you drink and the foods you eat. This includes fruits, vegetables, and even some meats you may consume. Each of these potentially replenishes some of the water that you MUST replace every day.

Here's the bad news: Extracting water from food and other beverages makes your body work harder – a lot harder – to get the water out, and more importantly obtaining water from food sources is usually not enough.

It all depends on what you eat and how fresh it is. Older, less fresh foods are more dried out. It also depends on the balance of what you eat. Do you eat a lot of fresh vegetables & juicy fruits? Or does your diet contain more bread, meats, cheese and other dairy?

The good rule of thumb is that everyone should add simple drinking water to your diet.

How Much Water Do I Need to Add, and How Should I Do It?

Some will advise adding over ½ gallon (64 ounces) of water per day over and above what you receive from your normal diet. Others will tell you adding 4 to 6 eight ounce glasses a day (32-48 ounces) is probably getting enough. BUT, rather than tell you a hard *"how much"* number I'm going to share with you a simple strategy that'll allow you to find out how much works for you.

Here it is: **For every cup or glass of milk, coffee, juice, beer, wine, or whatever you drink, follow it up with the same amount of pure water.**

If you drink one cup of coffee, drink one cup of water. Drink the additional cups of water before or after your coffee (I prefer drinking this additional water before my coffee). For every glass of wine you drink, immediately follow it up with one glass of water. This is an old trick I learned from wine lovers who say this helps each glass of wine taste better and also helps you stay sober longer (so they say!).

I follow this strategy and I drink even more water on top of that. But that's me. Over time, this strategy helped me discover that I'm in less pain when I consistently drink more water. Also, this simple "add a glass of water" strategy helped me figure out how to integrate the right amount of water into my life.

As a Bonus, Try Drinking Warm Water

Also, try drinking warm – almost hot – water all by itself. This is an Ayurvedic tip that can help you lose weight, improve digestion and is reportedly good for blood and lymph circulation. And, because it's relaxing to the entire body, drinking warm water helps to reduce pain in the body. This is my personal experience.

I highly recommend that you try this after a meal and also try it before your first cup of coffee in the morning. I think you'll be pleasantly surprised. If you're out for an evening on the town or have had a big meal and a few drinks, ordering plain hot water from your server will probably raise eyebrows but having a cup or two will be a blessing you'll remember. Try it!

What's More Important than Drinking Water? *Absorbing It!*

If you've never been a water drinker or you're a person who *never* drinks plain water I would advise you to start off slow. You've been getting water anyway through some of the foods you eat and other beverages you drink but, in this case, your cells have adapted to a more dried-out ecology. If you fit this profile and suddenly start pouring more water inside it's going to be like rain falling on hard parched earth – at first it's just going to run off until it starts to penetrate the deeper layers.

The objective is not to make our tissues and cells simply more "wet," but to make them more efficient – which will allow all of your systems to operate better and will hopefully reduce pain levels in your body. This is even more important if you're in chronic pain.

Here is where we could get into longer discussions on proper nutrition, PH levels and salt levels. But that is beyond the scope of this book. Instead, I'm going to suggest you follow the easy way outlined above to add water to your diet and your life – a cup or glass at a time.

Water is Not Just for Pain Relief – It's a KEY for Wellness

Relief from pain is only one part of living a life of better health and Wellness. You want your whole system to operate better which requires all the many systems in the body to interact with each other in a more optimal way.

Creating balance in your body is *key.* Having balanced hydration of all the cells and tissues in your body is *key.* Having balanced hydration – or not – directly impacts the effectiveness of all the other elements of your toolkit.

There's an old saying, *"If you pull one leg of the table the other three come along."* Discovering your right balance of water intake invites many other potential Wellness benefits to come along.

c. *The Gravity Pal*® Inversion Method™
and Other Customer Services

I've made it no secret that a big reason I wrote this book was to promote my Gravity Pal® low angle inversion tables. I hope that many of you will purchase one and take advantage of our 30-day risk-free trial offer where we even pay the shipping back to us if you decide that Gravity Pal® is not for you.[38]

In Chapter 8, I briefly outlined the *Gravity Pal Inversion Method™*. This gave you a feel for the basic elements of it. But there's a whole lot more to it.

Our customers receive a booklet (or a digital PDF) that we do not provide to the general public. This booklet is titled *"The Gravity Pal Inversion Method™ & Other Useful Information."* It is sent free – and exclusively to – those who purchase our Gravity Pal® low angle inversion tables.

I mention this because it is the gateway to the services we provide of which I hope you'll want to take advantage. Here is an outline of what we cover in that booklet:

---

[38] Conditions apply. Go to: http://www.gravitypal.com/wp-content/uploads/2016/04/Gravity-Pal-Warranty-30-Day-Risk-Free-Trial-Free-Return-Policy-PDF.pdf

1. Gravity Pal® Quick Start Guide. Provides the Right & Wrong Way to Get On and Off
2. The Importance of Resting After Your Gravity Pal® Sessions
3. Tips for using your Gravity Pal®
4. Tips for Integrating your Gravity Pal® Sessions into Your Daily Life
5. The Value of Shorter 1 to 3 Minute Sessions versus Longer Sessions
6. Special Things To Do On A Gravity Pal® I've Found Useful For:
    a. Low Back Tension
    b. Hips
    c. Mid-Back
    d. Shoulders & Neck
    e. Head
7. Frequently Asked Questions

We also provide ongoing support and valuable information to our customers from time to time.

Here's a Taste

A few pages ahead, in Appendix III we present our *Invitation to Researchers.* As you read that section you will see links for several articles that connect the Wellness side-benefits people have reported using their Gravity Pal® low angle inversion tables.

On our website, Facebook and YouTube pages you will also find other valuable articles. Occasionally you'll be introduced to fascinating authors and Self-Care authorities who specialize in many areas from Pain Management, Ayurveda to Trauma Release – plus many other topics.

Two examples of these fascinating authorities are Dr. Jacob Teitelbaum, an expert on Pain Management, and Dr. Peter A. Levine who is a Trauma Release specialist.

As I write this, I am in the process of arranging an interview with Dr. Teitelbaum, which I'm sure you'll enjoy.

Dr. Levine started a whole new approach at releasing trauma with his first book, *Waking the Tiger: Healing Trauma* when it was released in 1997. Below are a few words about both of these fascinating and illuminating people.

Dr. Jacob Teitelbaum – Pain Management

Dr. Teitelbaum, M.D. is a board certified internist who appears often as a guest on news and talk shows nationwide including Good Morning America, the Dr. Oz Show, Oprah & Friends, CNN, and Fox News Health. He's known for his breakthrough work on relieving the pain and fatigue experienced by those with fibromyalgia.

Dr. Teitelbaum has several best-selling books, provides an online evaluation service, and has promoted a natural pain relieving, anti-inflammation herbal supplement called *Curamin* that I personally use and endorse. For me, *Curamin* has been a godsend.

He is also a personal friend. I asked Dr. Teitelbaum to have his staff send me a few words summarizing his approach to pain relief and pain management we could include in this book. You will notice he mentions my Gravity Pal® low angle inversion table, which was a happy surprise to me.

Disclosure: *I do not have any financial arrangement with Dr. Teitelbaum for his comments on Gravity Pal®. He owns one himself and his comments are from his experience.*

From Dr. Teitelbaum:

"Got pain? One simple understanding can change your life. Pain is not an outside invader like infections. Rather, it is part of your body's monitoring system telling you something needs attention, like the oil light on your dashboard. Just like putting oil in the car makes the oil light go out, giving your body what it needs makes the pain go away.

This was demonstrated in our published fibromyalgia study about optimizing energy production with our S.H.I.N.E.® protocol that includes: Sleep, Hormones, Inflammation, Nutrition, and Exercise.

In our published study, S.H.I.N.E.® resulted in an average 91% improvement.

*The problem we all share? None of us were given an owner's manual for our body to tell you what the kind of pain you're experiencing means. **To remedy this, simply get the free phone app "Cures A-Z",** which discusses each kind of pain and how to remedy it.*

For back and muscle pain, this usually represents low energy in the muscles, and S.H.I.N.E.® helps.

*I invite you to try the **free** Energy Analysis Program at **www. EndFatigue.com** that can tailor a protocol to your case.*

As you restore energy production, you will find the Gravity Pal® low angle inversion table to be increasingly effective.

Meanwhile, for most kinds of pain, a special herbal mix called Curamin can be a pain relief miracle. Give it six weeks to see the full effect." [39]

---

[39] Learn more at www.EndFatigue.com

<u>Dr. Peter A. Levine</u>

Peter Levine, Ph.D. is the originator and developer of *Somatic Experiencing*® and the Director of the Foundation for Human Enrichment which you can read more about at https://traumahealing.org.

Dr. Levine holds doctoral degrees in both Medical Biophysics and Psychology. During his nearly fifty years of studying stress and trauma, he has contributed to a variety of scientific, medical, and popular publications. His book, *Waking the Tiger: Healing Trauma* is in its fifth printing and has received wide international attention.

His basic – and revolutionary – premise is that traumas – whether physical or emotional, and whether initiated by sudden, impactful moments or experienced gradually over time – create a situation where the trauma "event" causes a *trapped traumatic energy which is stored within our body and we find difficult to release.*

His unique observation is that we should not try to relive traumatic events, but simply get in touch with this blocked and stored energy and, through techniques he has developed, to release the energy *behind* the trauma.

His revolutionary insights have influenced many therapeutic approaches and modalities. I recommend that everyone read his books and watch the various YouTube videos interviewing him.

The above summaries will give you a taste of the kind of material that I continue to research and with which I am fascinated.

Please consider purchasing a Gravity Pal® so we can provide these additional services to you.

You can learn more about Gravity Pal® low angle inversion tables at www.GravityPal.com, and you can email me directly at mmckay@GravityPal.com.

Please watch our videos on Facebook and YouTube.

And please like us on Facebook at https://www.facebook.com/GravityPal

APPENDIX II

II. Resource Guide

    a. **Modalities I Regularly Use and Recommend**
    b. **Useful Websites & Books**
    c. **Tools I Have Found Useful**

a. Modalities I Regularly Use and Recommend

Transcendental Meditation Technique, www.tm.org

I have practiced TM for 20 minutes twice a day, every day since March of 1971 and, hands down, it is the most valuable modality I can recommend to anyone. The range of its scientifically verified effects is enormous, from stress management and PTSD recovery for veterans and others who suffer from traumatic stress, to improving the overall functioning of the brain, nervous system and cognitive abilities. Furthermore, TM is the only form of meditation to receive an endorsement from the American Heart Association as a treatment for high blood pressure and hypertension.

"A new report from the American Heart Association published on April 22, 2013 concluded that the Transcendental Meditation (TM) technique lowers blood pressure and recommends that the TM technique may be considered in clinical practice for the prevention and treatment of hypertension.

The purpose of the report, entitled "Beyond Medications and Diet Alternative Approaches to Lowering Blood Pressure: A Scientific Statement From the American Heart Association," *is to inform physicians which alternative approaches to lowering blood pressure (BP) have been shown by research to be effective.*

After considering meta-analyses and the latest clinical trials on different types of meditation, the report stated that while the Transcendental Meditation technique is recommended to lower BP, there is not enough scientific evidence to recommend other meditation or relaxation techniques." [40]

TM is not a religion, nor does it require that you follow a lifestyle. **Most importantly to me, you don't have to believe in it.** It's simply a technique and will work if it's properly done whether you believe it will or not. A TM session takes 20 minutes morning and evening and my experience is that the few minutes required adds *hours* of productivity to each of my days – not to mention all the other cumulative Wellness benefits I've derived. The instruction comes with a satisfaction guarantee and lifetime follow-up program wherever you may live.

Of all the modalities you can evaluate, this is the first one I believe everyone should try. It is absolutely the best investment – of any kind – I've ever made and delivers the most comprehensive positive effects on my life overall. **My Highest Recommendation**

Zero Balancing, www.ZeroBalancing.org

ZB is a hands-on modality that effectively balances both the structural and energy aspects of the body – at the same time. It is a clothes-on modality and takes less than an hour for a session.

Because I mentioned the word "energy" I would like to clarify that point. There are several different "energies" we commonly refer to in our human experience: mental energy, emotional energy, physical energy, and even conductivity throughout the nervous system, for example. We can experience imbalances in each of these aspects of energy. All of us have had the direct experience of this happening

---

[40] http://www.tm.org/blog/research/
american-heart-association-informs-doctors-tm-lowers-blood-pressure

from time to time; we all have more or less – sometimes a lot less – of each.

We can call these *aspects* of our personal life energy, which in Chinese medicine is called Chi (CHEE). From the Chinese perspective our energies – or Chi – can be blocked from flowing properly, and when that happens one of these aspects shows up as either depleted (weakened) or simply blocked.

Zero Balancing is a gentle, refreshing, and very practical modality that can bring balance to all of the various energetic aspects of a person, while simultaneously bringing balance to the physical, structural component parts of the human body. After receiving a ZB session you are likely to feel "new," "centered," and "balanced." For many people, it is a new kind of experience and defies easy description. The best single word is *integrative.*

It's that big.

Usually, a Certified ZB Practitioner is also certified in another dimension of bodywork or therapy that's primary focus is the structural aspect of the body, like massage, Rolfing, chiropractic or another medical training. I was introduced to ZB by my M.D., Dr. Jim Brooks, who was working to obtain his certification in ZB at that time.

A funny, true story: I came home after my first ZB session with Dr. Brooks and excitedly told my wife,

"I just had the most amazing experience – it's called Zero Balancing and you just have to try it!"

To which my wife said … firmly and with a wry smile,

"YOU NEVER LISTEN TO ME. I'VE BEEN TELLING YOU ABOUT ZB FOR TWO YEARS NOW!"

We laugh about that story now even though I'm a bit embarrassed to tell it. Fortunately, it has a happy ending.

I was so impressed with the results I obtained – and my wife was so delighted with the experiences that she was having – that both of us went through the training to be certified in ZB. We also, as a result of starting the ZB training, decided to go to massage school to become licensed massage therapists, as well. For us, we initially just wanted to take care of each other better – and wanted to obtain the training to be able to do so.

I can't say enough about ZB. It's an awesome, elegant, and practical modality that effectively helps one to *quickly* regain balance. ZB can help a person in so many ways. It can help unravel deeply rooted physical blocks. It is also very effective in releasing trauma from the body.

During the chaotic days following 9-11 in New York City, a few Zero Balancing practitioners devoted many 8-hour days giving ZB sessions to traumatized emergency response workers. There have been other ZB practitioners who have teamed up with doctors to assist people with various other trauma-related conditions, from emotional abuse to brain concussions.

I wish everyone would learn this modality for themselves and the people they most care about. Please check out Zero Balancing and find a practitioner in your area to get started.

<u>Massage</u>

My wife and I are licensed massage therapists. I love massage and receive one once a week. I recommend it to everyone and have been routinely receiving them since the 1970s. Regularly receiving massage can reduce pain, stress, muscle tension – and many other benefits as well.

The *American Massage Therapy Association's* web page lists *"25 Reasons to Get a Massage"* and provides links to many scientific studies where you can learn more.[41]

It's said that Hollywood legend Bob Hope, who lived to be 100 years old, received a massage every day for 63 years and fervently believed in the therapeutic benefits of massage.

Massage is a gift that you give to yourself. Receiving massage regularly is a great habit to start and one you will look forward to. Make sure your massage therapist is either licensed in their state or has graduated from a credentialed school – requirements vary from state to state. Avoid those not properly credentialed. Ask your doctor or chiropractor for a few referrals.

Also, question massage therapists closely on what modalities they've been trained in and like to use, and ask them to describe what receiving a massage from them FEELS like. Personally, what I don't want is someone whose touch is so light my tissues are not being "moved" (it feels to me like I'm being tickled) or that they use so much force (with a bony elbow or knuckle) that it's too uncomfortable.

But that's me. You might like that. So, ask before you make the appointment.

---

[41] *"25 Reasons to Get a Massage"*
   https://www.amtamassage.org/articles/1/News/detail/3124

If at all possible, find a massage therapist who is also trained in Myofascial Release Therapy[42] and Zero Balancing.

There are several schools of Myofascial Release but they all focus on the same thing – releasing deeper layers of adhesions, or "stuck points," in a very effective way. If you have localized areas that are constantly bothering you this kind of therapeutic approach can significantly help.

I've already talked about Zero Balancing before, but now is the time to bring out one more important aspect to it. ZB certification includes an important training in how to *calibrate* touch to the person receiving the session that goes far beyond any other training of which I'm aware. There is a *profound* layer of sensitivity that is taught and required with ZB that when applied to massage, makes massage a better experience. This is not to say that other professional and properly credentialed massage therapists cannot also have sensitivity but, if you're new to massage, I would recommend you find a massage therapist who also has that faculty refined by the certification training in Zero Balancing.

Five Element Acupuncture, https://WorsleyInstitute.com

Dr. Jim Brooks, who introduced me to Zero Balancing, also introduced me to *Five Element Acupuncture* which is a unique approach to acupuncture focused on restoring systemic balance to the individual. As such, it is squarely aligned with the message of *The Inversion Revolution:* to focus on balance and regaining balance. It complements Zero Balancing beautifully. I recommend it.

---

[42] *Learn more about Myofascial Release at https://www.spine-health.com/treatment/ physical-therapy/myofascial-release-therapy*

Weight Training

I'm partial to weight bearing exercises because, if approached properly, they strengthen the various fibers of the body: muscle, ligament, tendon and bone. Stronger fibers – in all the various forms they are seen throughout the body – in my opinion are fundamental to good health. This does not mean that you have to sign on to become a "weightlifter" or get into body sculpting. It's about creating the best health *ecosystem* for yourself.

I mentioned in the discussion about drinking water that we are made up of "wet gooey stuff." Some "stuff" is more liquid-wet and other "stuff" is more solid-wet. Remember I told you that all of the various *functions* of the body all require a proper balance of this "wet gooey stuff."

Well, the fibers of the body are more solid-wet, and all the various functions of the body require them working well together. Just like drinking – and absorbing – the right balance of water will assist you in maintaining and regaining balance, so too keeping all the fibers in the body's matrix toned and working well supports you from top to bottom. Even a gentle use of light weights, used regularly, can help.

If you don't know how to start, go to a public gym and find out who the private trainers are. Tell them your goals – take note that your goals may change from time to time. Mine have varied in emphasis over the years.

Here are my goals *all the time:*

1. **Reducing Pain**

2. **Regaining Balance**

3. **Having Good Flexibility & Muscle Tone**

Here are different goals I've had from time to time with my weight training program:

1. **Getting ready for a Rock Climbing trip** by a certain date

2. **Being able to do 10 dead-hang pullups** by a certain date

3. **Improving Functionality in various ways** – Here, give examples of what improved functionality would look like for you, like increasing your grip-strength, or being able to take a walk without it hurting your hips.

It's important your weight trainer is an expert in two things: how all the muscles in the body interact with other muscles, and nutrition. You don't necessarily need to have your trainer design a whole diet program for you. But they should be able to watch two things that they understand deeply:

A. How your muscles are *interacting.* My experience is that small supporting muscles are often injured when only bigger muscles are the focus. You want a trainer whose knowledge of the human anatomy is so detailed that he or she can instantly see which muscles are being overtaxed if your form is incorrect, or even if your form *is* correct. It takes a trained eye to see that level of detail.

B. Nutrition. You need someone who will look at how you're working out and can estimate that you're undernourished in X and over-consuming in Y. That kind of trainer can help you modify your diet so that you're making the progress you want and need to reach your goals.

Another thing: don't go along with anyone who wants you to work out every day or 5 to 6 days per week. Your body needs to rest and recover between workouts. The older you are, the more sensitive you should be to this fact of life. If you work out (what for you is) too often you'll burn out and most likely hurt yourself along the way. The maximum workouts I recommend are 3 per week, and I recommend only 1 or 2 per week when a person is starting out.

I *strongly* recommend a warm Dead Sea Salt bath after every workout. It will reduce your soreness and hasten your recovery. Also, I strongly recommend 1 to 3 minutes on a Gravity Pal® low angle inversion table after every workout to also aid in the recovery process. You'll be glad you take these recommendations.

Weight training, done correctly can provide many Wellness benefits. Always start slow and when you start out do LESS than your upper capacity until after you've been regularly practicing weight training. Then, testing the upper edges is not only valuable, it's where you'll make real progress.

Chiropractic

Here's an old joke: *"How many chiropractors does it take to screw in a lightbulb?"*

Answer: *"One, but it requires six visits!"*

I love chiropractic. I think it gets a bad rap, as depicted in this joke.

Too often I see people using chiropractic to mostly *"get out the kinks."* If you approach chiropractic that way then, of course, you're going to resent it if you're told you should come back several times.

In my opinion, chiropractic, for many people, can be a cornerstone of their Self-Care program. However, here is where it gets very dicey because out of the 45,000 chiropractors in the USA today, it is very hard to find those that, in my opinion, are the kind you may want.

True fact: many of my best friends are chiropractors. However, after seeing umpteen of them over the course of nearly 50 years, I can tell you that I've met some fabulous ones and some – well – let's just say I'd rather we'd never met!

Here is my advice about picking a chiropractor. First, please read the book, *Medical Intimacy, Deeper Understanding Allows for Deeper Healing* by my dear friend and personal chiropractor, Dr. Charles Coram.[43] When you read it you'll get a clear picture what you want your chiropractor to be like. After you've read Dr. Coram's book, go and meet different chiropractors who've been recommended to you and see how they measure up to that image.

There are great chiropractors out there. This will help you find one that can be a terrific member of your team.

b.   Useful Websites & Books

<u>Ayurvedic Discussion on the Six Stages of Disease</u>
http://www.mapi.com/ayurvedic-knowledge/immunity/
ayurvedic-understanding-of-disease.html#gsc.tab=0

<u>Fascia and Connective Tissue:</u>
Myers, Thomas, *Anatomy Trains,* https://www.anatomytrains.com

<u>Longevity</u>
www.GrowingBolder.com

<u>Medical News, Education & Latest Research</u>
http://www.medicalnewstoday.com/

---

[43] *Medical Intimacy, Deeper Understanding Allows for Deeper Healing,* Dr. Charles Coram, Balboa Press, ISBN: 9781504375245 http://www.balboapress.com/bookstore/bookdetail.aspx?bookid=SKU-001093218

<u>Medical Commentary</u>

Dr. Michel Accad, M.D., blogs at *http://alertandoriented.com*

Medical Intimacy, Deeper Understanding Allows for Deeper Healing, Dr. Charles Coram D.C. *Balboa Press, ISBN: 9781504375245 http://www.balboapress.com/bookstore/ bookdetail.aspx?bookid=SKU-001093218*

***Reflections on Maharishi AyurVeda and Mental Health,* Dr. James Brooks, M.D.**

http://www.mumpress.com/books/reflections-on-maharishi-ayurveda-and-mental-health.html

***The Fatigue and Fibromyalgia Solution: The Essential Guide to Overcoming Chronic Fatigue and Fibromyalgia, Made Easy!,* Dr. Jacob Teitelbaum M.D.**

https://www.amazon.com/Fatigue-Fibromyalgia-Solution-Essential-Overcoming/dp/1583335145

***Your Brain is a River Not a Rock,* Travis, Frederick, Ph.D.,**

ISBN-13: 978-1469937212

https://www.amazon.com/Your-Brain-River-Not-Rock/dp/1469937212

***Growing Old is Not for Sissies,* Etta Clark,** Pomegranate, August 1986, http://www.ettaclark.com

https://www.amazon.com/Growing-Old-Not-Sissies-Portraits/dp/0876540582

***The Gravity Guiding System,* Dr. Robert M. Martin, M.D.,**

ISBN: 9780876540589

Bodyweight Exercises for Extraordinary Strength, **Johnson, Brad**
https://www.amazon.com/Bodyweight-Exercises-Extraordinary-
Strength-Johnson/dp/0926888781

c. Tools I Have Found Useful

Dead Sea Salt Baths http://deadseawarehouse.com

Q-Flex https://getqflex.com & **TheraCane** http://www.theracane.com

Gyrotonic Machine www.Gyrotonic.com

It should be mentioned again that Gyrotonics is a *modality* that
initially requires the supervision and instruction of a specially
trained and certified instructor. The Gyrotonic machine is a tool but
is not useful until you receive training for it. Use the website to find
a Gyrotonic instructor in your area to begin.

ROM Range of Motion Machine www.romquickgym.com

<u>**Please Note**</u>
*Discuss the use of the listed resources with your primary health care
professional before using any of them. Neither the author nor the
publisher accepts any liability as a result of following the advice
of any resource, nor injury from any resource, modality, or tool
mentioned.*

*As of August, 2017 the author does not have a financial relationship
with any resource or tool manufacture mentioned. The author
reserves the right to be paid for endorsement of any product in the
future, without notice.*

APPENDIX III

III. Invitation to Researchers

My wife and I are both licensed health professionals who believe in helping people help themselves, what we call Self-Care. We also try to be very careful with the claims we make experienced.

Many people have reported benefits, as presented in this book and on our website, but there exists virtually no scientific research on the topic of inversion in general.

And there exists none at all, that we've been able to find, on the relative merits of low angle inversion, or "slanting" as it is sometimes called, versus higher angle inversion, or by itself.

Even though we believe we have justifiable reasons to recommend low angle inversion, we readily acknowledge that many people have benefited from other ways to alleviate the compressive effects of gravity including inversion tables, inversion chairs and decompression tables. We are not attempting to debate that people should not use these methods, although it is clear that many people should avoid them for various reasons.

Instead, we believe we should present the rationales for low angle inversion and respect what method(s) people find working best for them. Indeed, we may find that some of these methods of seeking relief from the compressive effects of gravity may work better in combination with each other rather than standing alone.

Having said that, we who make and use Gravity Pal® low angle inversion tables have an admitted prejudice toward low angle inversion and believe that:

- ❖ Gravity Pal® low angle inversion tables deliver a more gentle approach that is easier for the body to, more immediately, start releasing muscle and fascial tension without the occurrence of "muscle guarding," which would inhibit the release of tensions,
- ❖ Because muscle guarding is kept to a minimum, shorter times of 2-3 minutes are very effective.
- ❖ It is easier for someone to fit in 2 or 3 minutes at a time, 2 or 3 times a day than to set aside 15 or 20 minutes for a session. Therefore, someone is more likely to make a habit of it and look forward to repeating the experience.
- ❖ Regular daily, short-duration sessions deliver positive cumulative effects.
- ❖ There is a spectrum of side-benefits that can be experienced from the regular, daily experience of low angle inversion. This spectrum of benefits can be quite large and can touch on a number of areas that contribute to better overall health and Wellness.
- ❖ Gravity Pal® low angle inversion tables are easy and comfortable to use to people of modest – or even lower – fitness levels. This dramatically expands the potential number of people who could use, and potentially benefit from, inversion.
- ❖ Finally, the *Gravity Pal Inversion Method™* is an important breakthrough that has broadened inversion's potential availability and use to people who otherwise are too old or infirm to even consider inversion.

We therefore make this invitation to researchers to examine the experiences we've reported and to determine through objective testing if these results can be independently verified.

Below we have listed some potential areas where formal research into low angle inversion could be – and in our opinion, should be – conducted.

Where available, links to articles are provided. These articles, in various cases, may further spur the justification for such research.

We hope that some researchers will contact us and start this research. We would like to help. However, we fully understand that we are in the business to make and sell Gravity Pal® low angle inversion tables and therefore researchers will want to be careful not to invalidate their research by working too closely with those, like us, who have a vested interested in seeing our theories and the experiences of our users validated.

To remedy this, we offer to supply Gravity Pal® low angle inversion tables – free of charge – to universities and medical research centers to conduct this needed research. We would give these units without any request for attribution or our participation – although we would quickly like to offer assistance if we can provide it. We ask only that valid, objective research methods be employed by serious professional researchers.

We know that many people suffer from compression-related ailments, and many more can potentially benefit from the broad spectrum of Wellness benefits that using Gravity Pal® low angle inversion tables and our *Gravity Pal Inversion Method™* can facilitate.

It is our most sincere hope that the work we are doing to bring Gravity Pal®, the *Gravity Pal Inversion Method™* and low angle inversion to the world will aid those who need it most.

Sincerely,
Michael McKay, LMT &
Dawn McKay, LMT, MS-SLP
Gravity Pal, Inc.
info@GravityPal.com | www.GravityPal.com

Suggested Areas of Research on Low Angle Inversion

- ❖ Brain Health & Increased Cranial Lymph Circulation
- ❖ Cognitive Function
- ❖ Joint and Spine Health
- ❖ Exercise Recovery
- ❖ General Health
- ❖ Method Efficacy & the *Gravity Pal Inversion Method*™

Brain Health & Increased Cranial Lymph Circulation – Implications and Questions

There is a perceived increase of blood flow and lymphatic fluid to the brain experienced during low angle inversion using a Gravity Pal®.

- ❖ What are the measurable changes in volume of blood and lymph?
- ❖ What are the implications?
- ❖ Could regular use lead to a reduction in Brain Bleeding (micro-bleeding) in the elderly? [44]
- ❖ Could regular use lead to a reduction in Brain Atrophy, normally associated with aging? [45]

There is a perceived increase of lymphatic fluid exchange throughout the body and within the head experienced during low angle inversion using a Gravity Pal®.

---

[44] *Study Finds Brain Bleeding is Common with Aging,* published November 11, 2010, http://www.medicalnewstoday.com/releases/207320.php , accessed August 24, 2015

[45] *Study warns of increasing incidence of brain bleeds in US population over the next 15 years,* published March 21, 2015, http://www.medicalnewstoday.com/ articles/291196.php , accessed August 24, 2015

❖ Is there a measurable increase of larger molecule waste removal in the brain via the lymphatic system? [46]

❖ If so, are there any implications and potential impacts on delaying, or eliminating, the onset of Alzheimer's Disease, MS, autoimmune disorders and Autism Spectrum? [47]

❖ Researchers have reported to the American Alzheimer's Association that exercise *"makes changes in the brain that could indicate improvements"*, and exercise *"could be a fountain of youth for the brain."* Furthermore, *"No currently approved medication can rival these effects [of exercise]."*

While exercise is being exhorted as valuable for brain health it is worthwhile to question what exact aspects of "exercise" are delivering these wondrous results. **Is it the increased blood and lymph flow to and from the brain that are delivering them?** It stands to reason. Blood delivers nutrients and oxygen, while the lymphatic system carries away the larger waste molecules for elimination.

If increased blood and lymph circulation is the reason exercise delivers these effects, it is a reasonable question to inquire if these same effects can be delivered *mechanistically.*

In the published article mentioned above, *Landmark Discovery of vessels connecting brain to immune system,* Professor Jonathan Kipnis, a professor in The University of Virginia's (UVa) Department of Neuroscience and director of UVa's Center for Brain Immunology and Glia, said the discovery

---

[46] *Landmark Discovery of vessels connecting brain to immune system*, published June 6, 2015, http://www.medicalnewstoday.com/articles/294965.php , accessed August 24, 2015

[47] Ibid

lymphatic architecture in the brain and cranium *"changes entirely the way we perceive the neuro-immune interaction. We always perceived it before as something esoteric that can't be studied. But now we can ask mechanistic questions."*

He states that we now can approach the problem of diseases in the brain *"mechanistically."*

Related to Alzheimer's Disease Professor Kipnis points to the buildup of protein in the brain that is characteristic of Alzheimer's, and suggests these clumps may be accumulating because they are not being efficiently removed by the lymphatic vessels.

It therefore seems appropriate to ask: ***could regular daily sessions of a few minutes on a Gravity Pal® low angle inversion table deliver similar results as aerobic exercise?*** [48]

Also regarding brain health, would regular use of low angle inversion using a Gravity Pal® be a strengthening method, whereby those with hypersensitivity to brain damage from minor head trauma could avoid chronic subdural hematoma (SDH)? [49]

Could regular sessions of low angle inversion strengthen the tissues throughout the brain and cranium? [50]

---

[48] *A Better Treatment for Alzheimer's: Exercise,* published August 4, 2015 NBC News,

[49] *Physical activity may protect older people from brain damage,* published March 12, 2015, *http://www.medicalnewstoday.com/articles/290675.php,* accessed August 24, 2015

[50] Ibid

Cognitive Function
Many users of Gravity Pal® low angle inversion tables report greater clarity of thinking and improved memory after only a few weeks of regular use. Why?

- ❖ Are there measurable levels of increased oxygen and nutrient infusion (via increased blood flow) into brain tissue during 1 to 3 minutes of a low angle inversion session?

- ❖ Are there longer-term effects of regular use of low angle inversion on maintaining brain volume? [51]

Joint and Spine Health

- ❖ What are the short and long-term impacts on those with chronic back or joint issues who regularly use a Gravity Pal® low angle inversion table?

- ❖ Can some scheduled back surgeries be postponed, or the need eliminated altogether, for those who regularly use a Gravity Pal® low angle inversion table? [52]

- ❖ Can there be an improvement in joint health, in particularly the shoulders and hips?

- ❖ What would be the mechanics?

- ❖ Is it that proprioceptive control is relaxed while resting on a Gravity Pal® low angle inversion table, and that this allows improved range of motion without muscle guarding?

---

[51] *Reduced Brain Volume May Predict Dementia in Healthy Elderly People,* published January 4, 2006, http://www.medicalnewstoday.com/releases/ 35648.php , accessed August 24, 2015

[52] NB: My first account answer to this question is a resounding YES. I was scheduled for back surgery and regular low angle inversion is the reason I was able to cancel it. Michael McKay, L.M.T.

Exercise Recovery

There have been many reports from users of Gravity Pal® low angle inversion tables who report recovering from vigorous physical activity more quickly by immediately getting on their Gravity Pal® low angle inversion table for as little as 3 minutes after playing sports, weight lifting or performing house or yard work.

- ❖ What are the mechanics and physiological processes behind these reports of shorter recovery times?

- ❖ Specifically, what physiological processes are speeded up, and why?

General Health

Stamina & Stress Relief

There are reports of a quickly-achieved, deep level of rest which is followed by improvements in energy stamina from regular users of Gravity Pal® low angle inversion tables.

- ❖ What is unique about the restfulness that is experienced on a Gravity Pal® low angle inversion table versus other forms of rest, like sleep?

- ❖ Is this a different form and level of rest and, if so, what are the specific metabolic differences, and what are the measurable changes in those metabolic processes?

Improved Skin Tone & Health
There are reports of improved skin tone from regular users of Gravity Pal® low angle inversion tables.

❖ What are the measurable changes in facial collagen improvement, and is it directly related to regular sessions of low angle inversion?

Digestion
There are reports of improved skin tone from regular users of Gravity Pal® low angle inversion tables.

❖ Could there be improvements in digestion due to regularly experienced compressive relief from gravity?

❖ Is stress in the body being progressively released by regular sessions of low angle inversion?

Method Efficacy & the *Gravity Pal Inversion Method*™
The *Gravity Pal Inversion Method*™ represents a new approach to inversion that heretofore the world has not seen.

❖ What are the short and long-term impacts of short duration (1 to 3 minutes at a time) and regularly experienced (2 to 3 times per day) sessions of low angle inversion using a Gravity Pal® versus irregular, sporadic use of Gravity Pal® low angle inversion?

❖ What are the comparative short-term and long-term effects of using the *Gravity Pal Inversion Method*™ with low angle inversion compared to using this method with high angle inversion?

❖ What are the comparative short-term and long-term effects of using the *Gravity Pal Inversion Method™* with low angle inversion compared to simply lying flat?

Researchers can contact Michael McKay at info@GravityPal.com

Acknowledgments

I've been lucky. The healers I've been blessed to discover had one thing in common; they encouraged me to not become dependent on them. Instead, in one way or another, they led me to understand that I, and only I, could become the General Contractor of my health.

Throughout this book I've acknowledged many of these great human beings. Some have written books I mention which I hope you'll find and read. Some are still practicing their craft and I hope some of you will avail yourself of their unique skills.

I want to take this moment to again acknowledge the key people in my Self-Care team: Dr. Jim Brooks, MD, Dr. Charles Coram, DC, John Worsfold, L.M.T. and Frederico Gama, Fitness Trainer. Every day I am grateful for my good luck to have found each of you.

My daughter Kelly McKay patiently and generously edited this book and taught me more than good grammar; she taught me how to collaborate. This book – and I – are better because of it.

Hundreds of Gravity Pal® customers have shared with me how using their Gravity Pal® has bettered their lives. They are the people who showed me the power of this tool and how using it in a particular way unlocks enormous advantages to their quality of life.

Many people have also kept me inspired in other ways to either make important advances or overcome the setbacks that always come with every worthwhile project. This list is long but there are a few I must thank. These include Ed Tiritilli, Henry Becker, Freeman Yoder, Emma Schwartz, Bryan Martin, John Marble and Paul Siemsen. None of this would have happened without your particular encouragement, wisdom, skill, knowledge and generosity.

Above all, I thank my wife, Dawn and daughters, Kelly and Marina. They continue every day to give me the purpose to overcome pain and obstacles and, especially, to celebrate Wellness in my life.

My gratitude to them is beyond words.